Paediatric Cardiology

An introduction

N. Archer and M. Burch

Paediatric Cardiology Unit
The John Radcliffe Hospital
Oxford
UK

With an additional contribution from
M. Runciman

CHAPMAN & HALL MEDICAL

London · Weinheim · New York · Tokyo · Melbourne · Madras

Published by Chapman & Hall, an imprint of Lippincott-Raven Publishers, 2–6 Boundary Row, London SE1 8HN, UK

Lippincott-Raven Publishers, 227 East Washington Square, Philadelphia, PA 19106-3720, USA

First edition 1998

© 1998 N. Archer and M. Burch

Typeset in 10.5/12 Sabon by Photoprint Typesetters, Torquay, Devon
Printed in Great Britain at the University Press, Cambridge

ISBN 0 412 73450 8

A catalogue record for this is available from the British Library

Library of Congress Catalog Card Number: 97-78092

Contents

Preface

Cardiac disease in children is common enough to present to doctors and nurses working in every area of children's health care but sufficiently unusual to be a source of anxiety and confusion to the generalist. The purpose of this book is to provide non-specialist paediatricians with a basis for dealing with the diagnosis and management of paediatric cardiac disease. This will enable them to refer children to a cardiac service in good condition and at the right time and also to be involved in follow-up in a general paediatric department. The information contained here should equip the reader with enough specialist knowledge to deal with many aspects of cardiac care in the district general hospital setting and to communicate well with the families of children with a cardiac diagnosis. The intention is that this book is practical and relevant for paediatricians including those in training and that it will also be helpful to specialist paediatric nurses.

We are grateful to many people who helped in the preparation, including Sandra Wells for secretarial help, Helen Greaves for providing ECG rhythm strips and our colleagues who have (sometimes unwittingly) been sounding boards for our ideas.

Nick Archer
Michael Burch
Oxford

Foreword

In recent years many specialities have advanced at a pace that can leave floundering those not privy to the arcane secrets of the craft. Cardiology is one such; just as one had got to grips with how to interpret an ECG, echocardiography and colour Doppler became the specialists' stock in trade. Genetic advances have been no less dramatic, the gene splitters pushing to one side those who prided themselves on diagnosing a syndrome by Gestalt.

It can be lonely in the general hospital out-patient clinic or special care baby unit, miles from the nearest expert on congenital heart disease or arrhythmias. The telephone, facsimile transmission and telemedicine links may be comforting but nothing beats the relief of having an authoritative textbook in the ward library. Michael Burch and Nick Archer are hands-on doctors who understand what paediatricians need to know when faced with a cyanosed newborn requiring urgent rescue by pharmacological duct preservation. Their chapters help consultants judge the optimum time to transfer a sick baby to the regional intensive care unit and nurses and paediatric trainees how to recognise the signs of cardiac decompensation.

As surgeons have become more daring, more and more children live on with bizarrely distorted cardiac plumbing. Their follow-up is necessarily within tertiary centres, but when they become acutely ill they may turn up on the doorstep of doctors unused to the complexities of their condition. Having Archer and Burch on tap will compensate for inexperience and isolation as it is the most practical of guides to children's heart disorders.

One more point: many doctors and scientists have great knowledge and skills. Not so many know how to communicate them. As editor of an international paediatric scientific journal, I often wonder why so many authors seem not to realise that what they write is of little value unless their readers can make sense of it. Praise be, Archer and Burch write in plain English. I recommend this eminently sensible and wise book to everyone responsible for looking after children with abnormal hearts.

Harvey Marcovitch
Department of Paediatrics
Horton General Hospital
Banbury
Oxfordshire
UK

Part One
General Topics

Cardiac assessment 1

Introduction

History taking and examination remain the foundations of evaluation of an infant or child with a suspected cardiac problem. The information obtained from these two activities allows a decision on the need for and urgency of further investigations. Some of these, such as echocardiography, are not available in all places where children with cardiac disease present; thus appropriate selection for timely referral is essential. Other investigations, namely electrocardiograph (ECG) and chest X-ray (CXR), are widely available but require expertise to be used effectively and a working knowledge of them is desirable for all paediatricians. Cardiac disease in childhood presents in a number of situations (Table 1.1) and application of the skills of history taking and examination will be modified to make them relevant to the circumstances.

Table 1.1 Presentations of cardiac problems

Fetus
- Diagnosis by echocardiography

Neonate and infant
- Heart failure, including hydrops
- Cyanosis
- Collapse
- Abnormal heart rate/rhythm
- Murmur
- Weak femoral pulses
- Dysmorphic
- Non-cardiac congenital abnormalities
- Abnormal weight gain – too slow, too fast

Older child
- Murmur
- Heart failure (acquired disease)
- Multisystem disease (e.g. rheumatic fever, Kawasaki's disease)
- Chest pain
- Palpitations
- Unusual episodes (collapse, giddiness)
- Syndrome diagnosed (e.g. Turner's, Marfan's, Noonan's)
- Hypertension
- Family screening

History   There are a number of areas to be covered.

GESTATIONAL

Exposure to possible teratogens and details of maternal disease may provide important aetiological clues (Chapter 3, p. 47). Increasingly, infants are born having had a fetal cardiac scan: it is very important to know both the indication and the result. A fetal heart scan abnormality must always be confirmed postnatally, a normal scan not necessarily so, but such a result should not be clung to if clinical assessment suggests a cardiac abnormality.

BIRTH HISTORY

Prematurity is a clue more to the presence of non-cardiac, especially respiratory, disease but may point to cardiac disease (patent ductus arteriosus). Birth weight can alert to a syndrome, for example congenital rubella if small for gestational age or maternal glucose intolerance if large. Birth asphyxia is associated with both persistent pulmonary hypertension and myocardial dysfunction.

FAMILY HISTORY

This is relevant not only because of recurrence risks, but also because many inherited or genetically determined conditions have cardiac components (Chapter 3). It may not be known that a particular condition is in the family until a newly or differently affected member is born; for example Noonan's syndrome, which is autosomal dominant, is often not diagnosed in a parent until a child with pulmonary stenosis presents. Sudden unexplained, particularly premature, death and atypical fits in the family should be enquired after. Functional as well as structural heart disease may be genetically determined, as in familial prolongation of the QT interval or Duchenne dystrophy and other muscular diseases.

CARDIAC SYMPTOMS

These may or may not be the presenting complaint. Questions need to be asked to clarify and enlarge each category and these will be considered under each heading. History and examination overlap frequently.

Cyanosis

Peripheral cyanosis is very common at all ages but particularly in the newborn period when, if it occurs without central cyanosis and with no apparent discomfort or ill health, it is normal. A blue/grey discoloration in the moustache area of young babies is often noted after feeding and, similarly, if not associated with any abnormal behaviour is not a cause for concern. Older children will have blue lips and extremities if cold and can look blue around the eyes as well as circumorally when vasodilated, for example after a hot bath. Changes in peripheral vasomotor tone in toddlers and young children are not associated with any symptoms but frequently cause anxiety in parents. Systemic arterial desaturation causing true central cyanosis can be difficult to recognize and if constantly present is frequently missed by parents and health-care workers. Episodic central cyanosis may be a sign of cardiac disease, as in hypercyanotic spells, or of respiratory or neurological disorders such as asthma, croup, apnoea and fits.

Respiratory symptoms

Breathlessness is the commonest respiratory symptom with a cardiac cause, its manifestation will vary with age. Poor feeding will characterize a breathless infant, reduced exercise tolerance will be seen in an older child; there are many other causes for these complaints. Large left-to-right shunts in infants will cause breathlessness, which can interfere with feeding even without definite heart failure being present. Pulmonary venous engorgement and pulmonary oedema in heart failure cause breathing difficulty at any age and in infants quite often grunting. Indrawing will often be noticed by parents and cold clammy sweatiness may accompany heart failure in infants. Stridor and wheeze may be due to airway compression either from abnormal vessels or vessel remnants as in vascular rings (p. 217) or from enlarged normal structures such as the left atrium in dilated cardiomyopathy (p. 99) and pulmonary artery in absent pulmonary valve syndrome (p. 221). Respiratory symptoms may be signs of associated abnormalities rather than directly attributable to cardiac disease such as tracheo- and bronchomalacia in conjunction with tracheo-oesophageal fistula. Cough can be caused by any of the causes of breathlessness but rarely predominates. Orthopnoea is occasionally reported by older children. Hoarseness can be a feature of dilated pulmonary arteries in primary pulmonary hypertension or may be postoperative, due to recurrent laryngeal nerve dysfunction.

Unusual episodes and chest pain

These may be neurological, respiratory, gastrointestinal or cardiac in origin and a detailed history is needed to help distinguish these causes

Table 1.2   Unusual episodes – points to determine in history

- Precipitant, warning, prodroma

- Relationship to exercise, posture, meals

- Details of attack
  - Sudden/gradual onset
  - Pain – where/type
  - Palpitations – tap out rate/rhythm
  - Breathing
  - Headache/giddiness/nausea

- Cessation
  - Sudden/gradual
  - Trigger e.g. vomit
  - Inducible (e.g. Valsalva)

- Family history of unusual episodes, fits, etc.

(Table 1.2). Cardiac causes include arrhythmias (Chapter 14), angina, effort syncope in left, or more rarely right ventricular outflow obstruction and hypercyanotic spells.

Cardiac pain is rare in childhood although chest pain is a common symptom and is usually explained by musculoskeletal problems, gastro-oesophageal reflux or anxiety. Children old enough to give a clear description of pain will have the features of pericardial or cardiac pain in pericarditis and myocarditis and sometimes in arrhythmias. Severe left ventricular outflow obstruction may cause angina but this is rare in childhood, as is effort syncope. Angina from coronary artery disease is presumably present in infants having pale, quiet, sweating episodes in association with anomalous origin of the left coronary artery from the pulmonary artery and may be seen acutely in or years after Kawasaki's disease. Sharp, usually left, chest pain that is neither clearly musculoskeletal nor clearly cardiac seems a characteristic of adolescents with haemodynamically trivial mitral valve prolapse.

Hypercyanotic episodes, commonly called blue spells or hypoxic spells, occur in people with dynamic pulmonary outflow obstruction and a ventriculoseptal defect, classically tetralogy of Fallot. They are rare in the newborn period. Typically they occur after crying, particularly on waking, when, instead of colour returning to normal after crying ceases, the infant or child remains very blue and is drowsy or even limp and unresponsive, with rapid and deep respiration. They should always be asked after in infants known or thought to have lesions at risk of spells and parents should be instructed to recognize and to know how to respond to them (p. 86). Hypercyanotic spells are a reason for urgent reassessment and treatment.

Poor weight gain

Acutely, heart failure will cause excessive weight gain through fluid retention, although this will very rarely be reported in the history. The exception to this is the newborn infant going into heart failure within 7–10 days of birth in whom poor feeding and an absence of the usual weight loss or even marked weight gain may have been noticed, although its sinister implications are rarely realized. Visible oedema may be reported in older children in heart failure. Cardiac disease is one cause of failure to thrive in infancy; usually, breathlessness or other cardiac symptoms are present. Lesions causing heart failure or at least increased lung blood flow are the ones likely to cause failure to thrive. Cyanosis as such does not affect feeding and weight gain significantly, although it may be present in patients who also have plethoric lungs or may be present in syndromes that involve constitutional or other reasons for small size. Older children with cardiac disease, usually acquired, may be anorexic and therefore lose weight, as in endocarditis and cardiomyopathy.

GENERAL ENQUIRY

Systematic review is important in history taking for any suspected condition. In the context of suspected congenital or acquired cardiac pathology it is part of the process of unearthing associated abnormalities or symptoms of multisystem diseases.

MEDICATION

A detailed drug history is important as drugs may cause cardiac symptoms (e.g. terfenadine may cause arrhythmias) or may delay diagnosis (e.g. when antibiotics partially treat endocarditis). Cough is a side effect of angiotensin converting enzyme inhibitors, which are increasingly used in children to treat heart failure and hypertension.

Examination

Details given here relate specifically to the cardiovascular system but of course all systems will be examined in detail in a patient presenting for the first time and information on more than one system is gathered simultaneously. The standard format of inspection, palpation, percussion and auscultation is given in Table 1.3 and is considered in detail below. Initial inspection should rapidly allow an idea of the severity of the illness to be obtained, so that necessary resuscitation is not delayed while detailed examination is carried out.

Table 1.3   Summary of features of cardiovascular examination

Inspection
- Dysmorphism
- Growth
- Acute/chronic ill health
- Cyanosis – central/peripheral/differential
- Clubbing
- JVP – height/waveform
- Chest or spine deformity
- Respiratory system noise/distress/symmetry
- Skin lesions

Palpation
- Pulse and pulses
- Suprasternal notch
- Precordium
- Trachea, chest expansion
- Liver size, spleen
- Oedema

Percussion
- Respiratory examination
- Liver size if unclear
- Ascites detection
- Precordial rarely useful

Auscultation
- Cranial
- Goitre/other swelling
- Abdominal/loin
- Respiratory
- Cardiac
  - Heart sounds
  - Added sounds
  - Murmurs
- Blood pressure

1. INSPECTION

Dysmorphic features may give important clues to an underlying unifying diagnosis as well as suggesting particular cardiac abnormalities to be considered. In a sick baby with cardiac disease it is easy to overlook dysmorphic features and it is also hard to look for others, for example ocular or palatal abnormalities. Any area not adequately examined must be documented and reviewed at the earliest appropriate time. Growth parameters are important at any age and may provide information on underlying diagnosis or duration and severity of illness.

Cyanosis has already been partly considered in the previous section, but there are additional points to consider on examination. Central cyanosis can be overlooked in those with a low haemoglobin concentration and wrongly suspected in polycythaemic newborn infants. Racial pigmentation can confuse at any age and petechiae on the face of a newborn can appear like cyanosis. Tongue colour should be checked if there is doubt: cyanosis here suggests oxygen saturation of less than 85%. Pink fingernail beds and blue toenail beds suggests right-to-left ductal shunting in a newborn, which may be due to persistent pulmonary hypertension or structural heart disease. In an older person this suggests elevated pulmonary vascular resistance (Eisenmenger's complex) with patent ductus arteriosus; often there will be clubbing of the toes in this situation. A baby with transposition and aortic arch interruption or severe coarctation will have less well saturated blood in the right hand than in the feet; this may be detectable clinically and is termed 'reversed differential cyanosis'.

Clubbing is not seen in the first year of life. It should be sought in upper and lower extremities (see above) and the largest available nails, thumbs and great toes, should be examined. Non-cardiac causes of clubbing should not be forgotten, particularly in the context of chronic ill health and suspected endocarditis.

The jugular venous pulse is difficult to see in babies and young children: they have short and often stocky necks, they do not lie still at 45° and they may have prominent external jugular veins. In addition the liver of young children is very distensible and changes size markedly with only small changes in central venous pressure. Thus for many reasons the height and waveform of the JVP are not studied under the age of 4–5 years. Thereafter, information can be gained from it just as in adults.

Chest and spine deformity should be looked for, as should signs of cardiac enlargement, chronic respiratory distress or associated skeletal abnormalities.

Respiratory rate, pattern, symmetry, indrawing and nasal flaring should be evaluated and expiratory grunting or other respiratory noises noted. These may reflect cardiac or respiratory disease. Skin lesions to be sought include rashes, as in Kawasaki's disease (p. 122) and rheumatic fever (p. 119), lesions of endocarditis (p. 113), features of collagen vascular diseases and markers for neurocutaneous syndromes.

2. PALPATION

Arterial pulses can be detected at radial, brachial, axillary, carotid, femoral, posterior tibial and dorsalis pedis positions. When general circulatory insufficiency is suspected a central pulse such as axillary or carotid should be confirmed and if detected more peripheral ones

Table 1.4   Information to be obtained from the pulse

- Rate
- Rhythm
- Volume
- Character

should be evaluated. Comparison of brachial or axillary and femoral pulses is important in the context of possible coarctation as also is comparing right and left arm and carotid pulses in judging possible arch interruption. Local arterial pathology, most commonly iatrogenic in children, is assessed by comparing peripheral pulses on each side, as well as by colour, temperature and capillary refill of the affected limb. Pulse information (Table 1.4) should be obtained from the most easily felt upper half artery usually right radial or brachial.

Suprasternal palpation is important: a thrill points to significant left ventricular outflow obstruction, usually aortic valve stenosis or less commonly patent ductus arteriosus, pulmonary stenosis and aortic arch abnormalities. Precordial palpation is to assess:

- apex position: 4th left intercostal space inside nipple under 5 years; 5th left intercostal space at or inside nipple over 5 years;
- apex character;
- presence of left parasternal heave, suggesting right ventricular hypertrophy;
- thrills: site and timing determined by underlying pathology.

Trachea position and symmetry of chest expansion are integral to the interpretation of observations made by suprasternal and precordial palpation.

Liver size should be assessed by palpation just lateral to the rectus muscle and reported in centimetres; the full contour of the liver should be assessed so as not to miss midline or predominantly left-sided livers. If palpation is inconclusive percussion may help, as may auscultation while gently scratching over the liver. Pulsation of the liver may be due to gross tricuspid regurgitation but must be distinguished from transmitted pulsation from the aorta, which is uncommon, or in young infants from the epigastric pulsation of right ventricular hypertrophy. Normal newborn infants may have 1 cm of liver palpable; in school-age children the liver edge can often just be felt below the costal margin. More liver than this can be felt if there is overexpansion of the chest, if right atrial pressure is elevated without heart failure as in tricuspid atresia or pulmonary atresia, and in heart failure. There are of course non-cardiorespiratory causes for hepatomegaly.

The spleen can just be felt in many newborns. A spleen felt on the right is to be expected in complete abdominal situs inversus. Splenomegaly must be distinguished from displacement by overinflation as in respiratory diseases. Ascites is rarely cardiac but can be a feature of severe heart failure in the fetus and newly born, as in hydrops fetalis, and is also seen in some patients with a Fontan-type circulation. Dependent peripheral oedema is a late sign of heart failure in children but should be sought over the sacrum and in the lower legs by firm and sustained pressure, which the child may find uncomfortable.

3. PERCUSSION

Percussion is an important part of respiratory examination but is rarely contributory or even necessary in obtaining cardiovascular information. It may help is assessing liver size and detecting ascites.

4. AUSCULTATION

Non-cardiac

A quiet systolic bruit over the anterior fontanelle is normal in infants; an intracranial bruit that is continuous and loud may point to an arteriovenous malformation as a cause of heart failure in an infant. Any possible vascular swelling should be auscultated to support the diagnosis of hyperaemia. Renal artery bruits and bruits from narrowing of the abdominal aorta are very rare in childhood. Crepitations and rhonchi in the chest can be a feature of pulmonary oedema.

Cardiac

The precordium should be listened to in the four cardinal areas and the back with both bell and diaphragm. When listening at the lower left sternal edge (tricuspid area) heart sound intensity should be compared with the right-hand side of the sternum; if louder in this latter position the possibility of dextrocardia should be considered by listening to the region of the right nipple and by palpating the precordium again.

It is important to be systematic in auscultation, concentrating on heart sounds, added sounds and murmurs in turn; it is also important to remember that many pathologies will have several abnormalities to hear. Particular auscultatory findings are given at the appropriate points in the text. Table 1.5 lists the features of murmurs to be sought.

5. BLOOD PRESSURE

Measurement of blood pressure is an integral part of cardiovascular examination and is important in the assessment of any baby or child

Table 1.5   Information to be ascertained about a murmur

● Timing	
Systolic	Early, mid, late, pan
Diastolic	Early, mid, late
Continuous	i.e. both sides of second sound
● Site and radiation	Neck
	Axilla
	Lateral chest
	Spine
● Loudness	Grade out of 6 (4 or more if a thrill)
● Quality	
● Variation with	Posture
	Respiration
	Valsalva/other manoeuvres

Table 1.6   Normal blood pressure: 90th and 95th centiles for blood pressure related to age (derived from: Report of the Second Task Force on Blood Pressure Control in Children (1987) *Pediatrics*, 79, 1–25)

Age (years)	1	3	5	8	10	12	15	18
90th centiles								
Girls								
Systolic	105	106	109	114	117	127	126	127
Diastolic	67	69	69	72	75	78	82	80
Boys								
Systolic	105	107	109	114	117	121	129	136
Diastolic	69	68	69	73	75	77	79	84
95th centiles								
Girls								
Systolic	109	110	112	117	121	125	130	132
Diastolic	71	72	72	76	79	80	86	86
Boys								
Systolic	109	111	115	117	122	127	133	140
Diastolic	72	72	74	76	79	80	84	89

Diastolic measurements are Korotkoff phase 4 (sounds become muffled), except at ages 12–18 years, when phase 5 is used (sounds disappear)
Normal blood pressure is defined as below the 90th centile; hypertension as on or above the 95th centile

presenting to medical attention, whatever the possible pathology. It should be measured in all cases in the right arm; in symptomatic infants and whenever coarctation is suspected it can be helpful to obtain measurements in the left arm and at least one leg.

Cuff selection is important: width should be approximately two-thirds of the distance from elbow to shoulder, or 50% of the arm diameter, the inflatable part of the cuff should reach almost all the way around the arm and the cuff size used should be documented. The same cuff can then be used on the calf; thigh cuffs should be assessed like arm cuffs and can be difficult to match in tall or obese subjects. If the cuff is too small a falsely high pressure will be obtained, just as it will if the child is crying or moving the limb. Similarly, an over-large cuff will under-read.

Pulse detection can be by auscultation, which will allow diastolic pressure to be measured, or by palpation or Doppler detection. The method used will affect results: palpation is less sensitive. The method used must be documented. Normal blood pressures are given in Table 1.6 and hypertension is defined as being above the 95th centile for age/height (p. 126). There is no demonstrated benefit in blood pressure screening child populations.

Investigations 2

History and examination should always precede investigation and will determine what, if any, investigations are required and the degree of urgency. Diagnosis of an innocent murmur after infancy does not necessarily involve any investigations. Many cardiac conditions can be diagnosed without tests, although most will be subject to investigation. A logical sequence of investigation is required and in many paediatric departments this will involve ECG and chest X-ray before ultrasound scanning, although this approach is being reviewed in many places with the increasing availability not only of suitable ultrasound equipment but also of appropriate expertise. In this section common investigative tools will be reviewed in turn. Details of findings in particular conditions will be found in the relevant chapters and in Part 5.

The ECG has been used in evaluating known and suspected cardiac disease in children for 80 years. It is of value in assessing rhythm and conduction disturbances as well as in helping to recognize chamber enlargement, hypertrophy and strain. The ECG is useful in following the progression of many structural abnormalities, it is readily available and does not require the expensive equipment and operator expertise of ultrasound scanning. Interpretation of the ECG must always take into account the child's age with reference to tables of normal values (Tables 2.1, 2.2).

An observer must be able to describe an ECG sequentially before interpretation can be reliably carried out. Lead positions are as for the standard adult ECG with the addition of V4r being recorded in children to give further assessment of the right heart (assuming a normal heart position). If the heart is predominantly in the right hemithorax leads V5r and V6r should also be recorded.

Table 2.1 Table of ECG normal values (ages 0–12 months)

	days				months		
	0–1	*1–3*	*3–7*	*7–30*	*1–3*	*3–6*	*6–12*
Heart rate (beats/min)	94–155	92–158	90–166	106–182	120–179	105–185	108–170
PR lead II (ms)	80–100	81–139	74–136	72–138	72–130	73–146	72–157
QRS duration (ms) VS	21–75	22–67	21–68	22–79	23–75	22–79	24–75
Frontal QRS axis (°)	+60 to +190	+62 to +196	+75 to +190	+65 to +160	+30 to +115	+5 to +105	+5 to +100
Q wave (mV)							
lead III	0–0.52	0–0.51	0–0.48	0–0.55	0–0.54	0–0.65	0–0.63
AVF	0–0.34	0–0.33	0–0.35	0–0.35	0–0.34	0–0.32	0–0.33
V1	0	0	0	0	0	0	0
V6	0–0.17	0–0.21	0–0.28	0 to 0.28	0–0.26	0–0.26	0–0.30
R wave (mV)							
V1	0.5–2.6	0.5–2.6	0.3–2.4	0.3–2.1	0.3–1.8	0.25–2	0.1–2
V6	0–1.1	0–1.2	0–1.2	0.25–1.6	0.5–2.1	0.6–2.25	0.6–2.3
S wave (mV)							
V1	0–2.3	0–2.1	0–1.7	0–1.1	0–1.25	0–1.7	0.01–1.8
V6	0–1.0	0–0.9	0–1.0	0–1.0	0–0.7	0–0.9	0–0.75
R/S							
V1	0.2–9.8	0.2–6	0.2–9.8	1–7	0.3–7.4	0.2–6	0.2–4
V6	0.2–10	0.2–11	0.2–10	0.2–12	0.2–12	0.2–18	0.2–21

P WAVES

P waves are due to atrial depolarization. Normal P waves have a frontal axis of 0° to +90°, are not more than 2.5 mm high and are of less than 120 ms duration. Abnormalities of P waves can be informative in the following circumstances.

- **Abnormal axis.** This means one of four possibilities:
  - not sinus rhythm (PR interval may also be short);
  - heart not in usual position;
  - atria not in normal spatial relationship;
  - leads transposed (examine V6, which should be similar in polarity to lead 1; if it is not, right arm and right leg leads have been exchanged).
- **P waves not all associated with QRS complexes or not all QRS complexes have P waves.** This means that a dysrhythmia or conduction disturbance of some sort is present (Chapter 14).

Table 2.2 Table of normal ECG values (ages 1–16 years)

Years	1–3	3–5	5–8	8–12	12–16
Heart rate (beats/min)	90–150	72–137	64–132	62–130	61–120
PR lead II (ms)	82–148	84–161	90–164	87–171	92–175
QRS duration (ms) V5	27–75	30–72	32–78	32–85	34–88
Frontal QRS axis (°)	+5 to +100	+5 to +105	+10 to +140	+5 to +115	+10 to 130
Q wave (mV)					
lead III	0–0.53	0–0.42	0–0.32	0–0.26	0–0.30
AVF	0–0.32	0–0.29	0–0.25	0–0.26	0–0.19
V1	0	0	0	0	0
V6	0–0.29	0–0.33	0–0.46	0–0.27	0–0.29
R wave (mV)					
V1	0.25–1.8	0.1–1.8	0.05–1.4	0.02–1.2	0.02–1
V6	0.6–2.3	0.8–2.4	0.8–2.7	0.9–2.6	0.7–2.3
S wave (mV)					
V1	0.05–2.1	0.15–2.2	0.3–2.3	0.3–2.5	0.3–2.1
V6	0–0.65	0–0.55	0–0.4	0–0.4	0–0.38
R/S					
V1	0–4	0–2.8	0–2	0–1.9	0–1.8
V6	0.2–27	0.3–30	0.3–30	1–33	1–39

- **Abnormal dimension:**
  - more than 2.5 mm tall reflects right atrial enlargement;
  - more than 120 ms in duration (may be notched or biphasic) signifies left atrial enlargement.

PR INTERVAL

This is measured from the start of the P wave to the start of the QRS complex; hence 'PQ interval' may be a more appropriate description. The PR interval varies with age and heart rate: normal values are given in Tables 2.1 and 2.2. The PR interval can be:

- **too short.** This suggests a pre-excitation pattern when anterograde conduction is occurring through an accessory atrioventricular pathway. Other features of pre-excitation should be sought carefully in the form of QRS prolongation with slurring on the upstroke of the R wave (see Figure 14.10). A short PR interval may also be found without pre-excitation in Pompe's disease and Duchenne muscular dystrophy, and if atrial impulses are arising from other than the sinus node.

- **too long.** This is first-degree heart block. It can be harmless and it may be due to drugs (e.g. digoxin) or intercurrent illness (acute feverish illnesses, including rheumatic fever, diphtheria, Lyme disease). First-degree heart block can be associated with structural heart disease, e.g. atrial septal defect (ASD), and can be familial. It may occur postoperatively. Isolated first-degree heart block in a structurally normal heart is usually considered harmless but may be a marker for the development of more serious and symptomatic degrees of heart block (Chapter 14).

THE QRS COMPLEX

This reflects ventricular depolarization. The following points are of practical importance.

Duration

This varies with age (Tables 2.1, 2.2). Abnormally long QRS duration means either bundle branch block (right or left, determined by morphology) or pre-excitation, in which case there is slurring of the R wave upstroke (delta wave), particularly in the chest leads (Figure 14.10). In pre-excitation a short PR interval is nearly always seen.

Frontal axis

The frontal axis (Figure 2.1) varies with age (Tables 2.1, 2.2) and should only be calculated on the initial portion (80 ms) in the presence of bundle branch block. An abnormal axis is helpful in a number of circumstances.

- **Right axis deviation** is commonly found in right ventricular hypertrophy.
- **Left axis deviation** may indicate left anterior hemiblock, which can be postoperative or is commonly seen in the following conditions:
  - ostium primum ASD (partial atrioventricular septal defect – AVSD);
  - tricuspid atresia;
  - pulmonary valve stenosis when the valve is dysplastic and the child has Noonan's syndrome.
- **Axis in the 'north west'** (Figure 2.2). This reflects right or extreme left axis deviation, is rarely normal and is an important marker for:
  - complete AVSD;
  - complex cardiac anomalies.

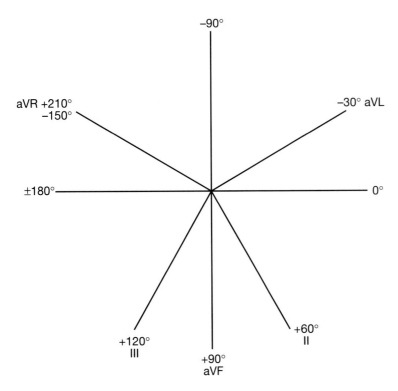

Figure 2.1   Hexaxial reference system. This diagram allows the frontal axis of the QRS complex (or P wave) to be determined. Depolarization directly towards an ECG lead produces a positive deflection on the trace; away produces a negative deflection. The lead at right angles to the direction of depolarization is equiphasic. In order to estimate the frontal axis: (1) Identify the most equiphasic lead. (2) The frontal axis will be at right angles (± 90°) to this lead. (3) Examine the leads at right angles; the one with a mainly positive deflection is the approximate frontal axis. (4) More precision can be obtained by 'imagining' the truly equiphasic position between leads and placing the axis at right angles to this. (5) If all leads are equiphasic or nearly so, the axis is said to be indeterminate.

QRS configuration

The following points are important.

- Q waves are not normal in right chest leads. They point to severe right ventricular hypertrophy (RVH), conduction disturbance (left bundle branch block or pre-excitation) or congenitally corrected TGA.
- Abnormally deep Q waves in leads 2, 3, V4–6 suggest septal or left ventricular hypertrophy.

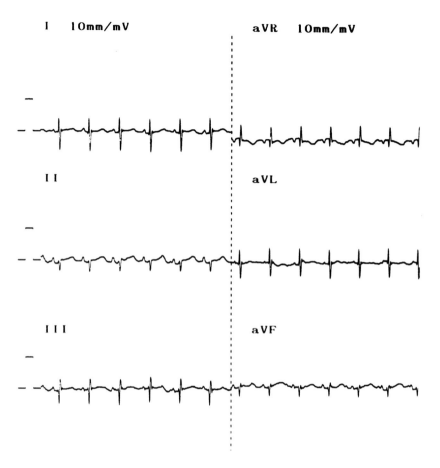

Figure 2.2   ECG example. Standard (I, II, III) and limb leads (aVR, aVL, aVF) on an infant showing 'north-west' QRS axis (aVL equiphasic, lead II predominantly negative making axis away from + 60°. (See Figure 2.1.)

- Abnormally large voltages indicate ventricular hypertrophy, the left ventricle being reflected by S waves in the right chest leads and R waves in the left chest and the opposite being the case for the right ventricle.

Ventricular hypertrophy is indicated by the following features.

- **Right ventricular hypertrophy:**
  - right axis deviation;
  - upright T wave in V1 after day 3 and under 6 years of age;
  - neonatal R/S progression across the chest leads after the newborn period (i.e. dominant R in V1 and dominant S in V6 – Figure 2.3);

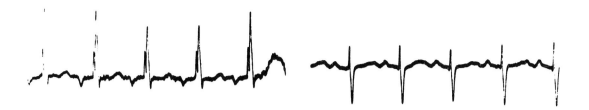

Figure 2.3   ECG example. Leads V1 and V6 showing a dominant R wave in V1 and a dominant S wave in V6, a neonatal R/S progression that is abnormal after 4 weeks of age. Note also the upright T wave in V1, normal in the first 48–72 hours of life but not thereafter until at least mid-childhood: before this, it indicates RVH.

  - abnormally large R wave in V1 or S in V6.
- **Left ventricular hypertrophy:**
  - adult R/S progression from lead V1 to V6 under 12 months of age (dominant SV1, dominant RV6 Figure 2.4);
  - abnormal left ventricular voltages RI, II, III, aVL, aVF, SV1, RV6 (Tables 2.1, 2.2).
- **Combined ventricular hypertrophy:**
  - combined features of the lists above;
  - large voltages in two or more standard leads and across mid-chest leads in an infant (Katz–Wachtel phenomenon).

ST SEGMENTS AND T WAVES

Changes in ST segment can reflect ischaemia (depression), digoxin therapy (depression), pericarditis (elevation) and myocardial infarction (elevation over affected areas with reciprocal depression in leads opposite the involved site).

Common or important T wave changes include:

- ischaemia, infarction and myocarditis cause inversion;
- conduction disturbances such as pre-excitation or bundle branch block cause abnormal polarity;
- hyperkalaemia causes peaked T waves, progressing to broadening of the QRS complex and bradycardia, with disappearance of P waves;
- flat T waves are seen in hypothyroidism, hypokalaemia, myocarditis and pericardial effusion; in pericardial effusion QRS complexes are of small voltage.

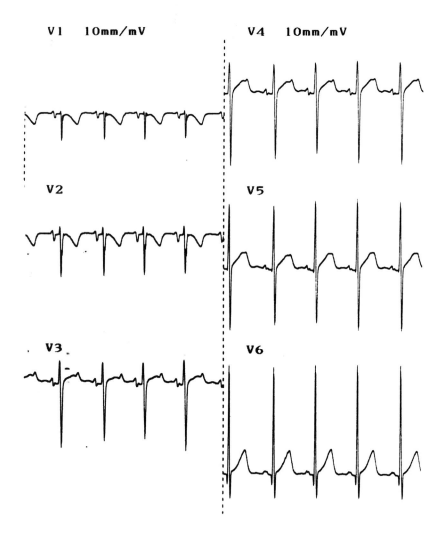

Figure 2.4 ECG example. Chest leads (V1–V6) showing a dominant S wave in V1 and a dominant R wave in V6, an adult R/S progression not normally clearly established until 18 months of age: before this it indicates LVH.

QT INTERVAL

This varies with heart rate and is usually adjusted for this by calculating the corrected QT interval (QT_c), which is discussed in detail in Chapter 14. Measurement of the QT interval when the heart rate is fast, the T wave is bifid or there are prominent U waves can be problematic. A long QT_c may be due to:

● drugs (e.g. quinidine, procainamide, disopyramide, amiodarone, sotalol and propafenone);

- hypocalcaemia;
- bundle branch block;
- myocarditis;
- prolonged QT syndromes, often familial, in which case they are frequently associated with serious ventricular arrhythmias (p. 161).

SPECIAL ECG MODALITIES

Ambulatory ECG monitoring can be useful in identifying arrhythmias or conduction disturbances and relating symptoms to the presence or absence of rhythm disturbances.

Cardiomemo devices are useful when intermittent but potentially serious symptoms occur, and consist of a device issued to the family for recording an ECG during an episode.

Exercise testing has a valuable role in a number of areas of paediatric cardiology, including occasionally looking for ischaemic changes, although investigation of possible arrhythmias and evaluation of exercise tolerance and blood pressure response to exercise are more usual reasons for the investigation in children.

Tilt table testing is a way of assessing sino-atrial function when syncope or near syncope is thought possibly to be due to unusual autonomic activity or abnormal sinus node responsiveness. It is widely used in adult cardiology and is becoming more commonly applied to older children. The subject is kept still in vertical or near-vertical position for varying lengths of time and changes in heart rate and blood pressure are recorded.

Chest X-ray

Chest X-ray (CXR) is widely used and, along with an ECG, is the time-honoured first step in investigating a child with suspected heart disease. In the initial work up of a newly presenting case it is indicated in the following circumstances.

- symptomatic neonate;
- asymptomatic neonate not thought to have an innocent murmur;
- in infancy and childhood if possible cardiac symptoms present;
- in infancy and childhood if a murmur is thought not to be innocent.

It should be noted that, particularly after infancy, a CXR does not aid in the discrimination between innocent and significant heart murmurs if the child is assessed by an experienced clinician. In infancy, including

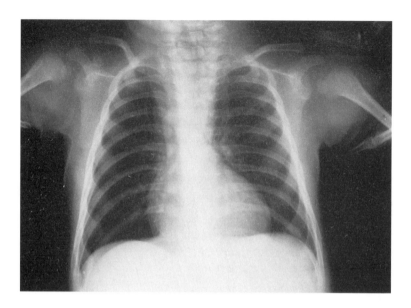

Figure 2.5   Postero-anterior chest X-ray. Left-sided heart and apex, normal heart size, aortic arch side not clear, stomach and liver position not clear. Central pulmonary artery small, lung fields oligaemic. Infant with tetralogy of Fallot.

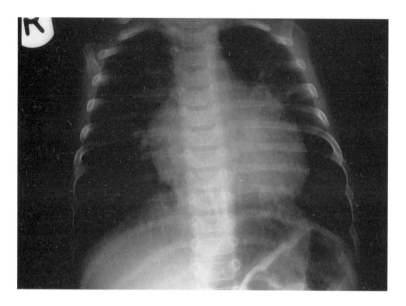

Figure 2.6   Postero-anterior chest X-ray. Left-sided heart and apex; stomach on left, liver on right. Enlarged heart shadow (cardiothoracic ratio above 60%) with pulmonary plethora. Infant with large VSD.

the newborn period, the same is probably true but the CXR remains widely used in the investigation of suspected innocent murmurs in the first year of life.

Points to look for on an X-ray done because of definite or suspected cardiac disease (Figures 2.5–2.8) are:

- **heart position**: left, right or central;
- **apex side**: left or right;
- **bronchial and abdominal situs**: usual, inverted, ambiguous;

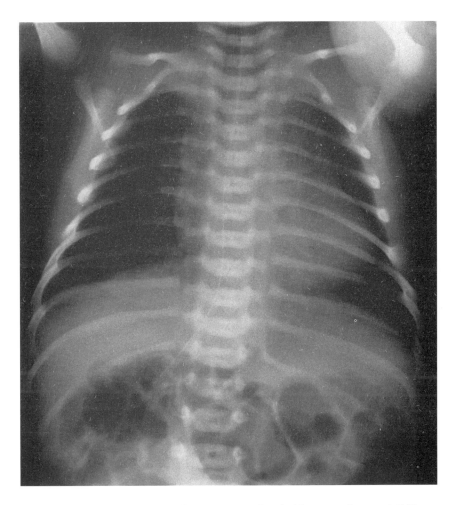

Figure 2.7 Postero-anterior chest X-ray. Left-sided heart and apex. Midline liver, right-sided stomach (with nasogastric tube), pointing to an abnormality of atrial situs and the strong possibility of cardiac disease. Infant with left-sided isomerism, VSD and subvalvar pulmonary stenosis.

- **aortic arch**: left- or right-sided, abnormal contour of ascending or descending aorta;
- **presence of thymus shadow**: frequently not obvious after newborn period;
- **heart size and contour**: cardiothoracic ratio up to 60% in normal infants, 50% thereafter;
- **pulmonary vascular markings**: increased or decreased;
- **abnormalities of the diaphragm**: abnormal elevation;
- **pulmonary pathology**: collapse/consolidation;
- **skeletal abnormalities**: spine and ribs especially.

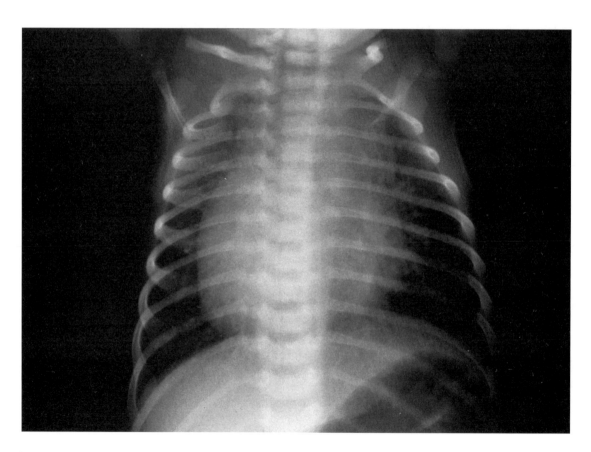

Figure 2.8 Postero-anterior chest X-ray. Right-sided heart and apex; stomach on left, liver on right. Unusual heart shape. Infant with two VSDs and pulmonary stenosis with no abnormality of atrial, visceral or bronchial situs.

Two-dimensional echocardiography was first introduced in the 1960s, but accelerated development in its clinical use occurred in the USA in the next decade. It would not be an overstatement to say that the technique has revolutionized the practice of paediatric cardiology. This painless, non-invasive technique is ideally suited to the investigation of congenital heart disease. It can be used at the bedside and in intensive care units. Many children will now go to the operating theatre principally on the basis of an echocardiographic assessment without resort to cardiac catheterization and angiography. The cardiac structures are nearer to the surface of the chest in children and therefore high-frequency (e.g. 5 MHz and 7.5 MHz) transducers can be used, which have poor penetration but good image resolution. In young adults the ultrasound windows are not as good and lower-frequency transducers are usually required, giving inferior resolution. Sometimes the images are so poor that transoesophageal echocardiography is used. This technique may also be appropriate in the operating theatre or in the intensive care unit when a traditional transthoracic scan cannot be performed, but many cardiac surgeons now perform intraoperative echocardiography by placing the transducer directly on the heart.

The real-time images produced by two-dimensional echo display cardiac anatomy clearly, whereas the images produced by M-mode echocardiography (which employs a single ultrasound beam looking at the change in time of a particular point in the heart) is useful for detailed measurements, for example to study ventricular function.

Examples of normal and abnormal ultrasound scans are shown in Figures 2.9–2.13.

DOPPLER ECHOCARDIOGRAPHY

The important principle for Doppler echocardiography is that the frequency of ultrasound changes when it is reflected from a moving target (Doppler shift) and this change is related to the speed of the target. If the frequency of the ultrasound being emitted is known then that of the beam received is detected. The Doppler shift can be displayed as a velocity (Figure 2.14). Most machines can convert this into a pressure gradient (using the modified Bernoulli formula), enabling the pressure gradient across the valves and VSDs to be determined.

COLOUR FLOW DOPPLER

Colour flow Doppler (Plate 1) displays a real-time image of flow across the valves. A colour 'map' is created, with segments of the map

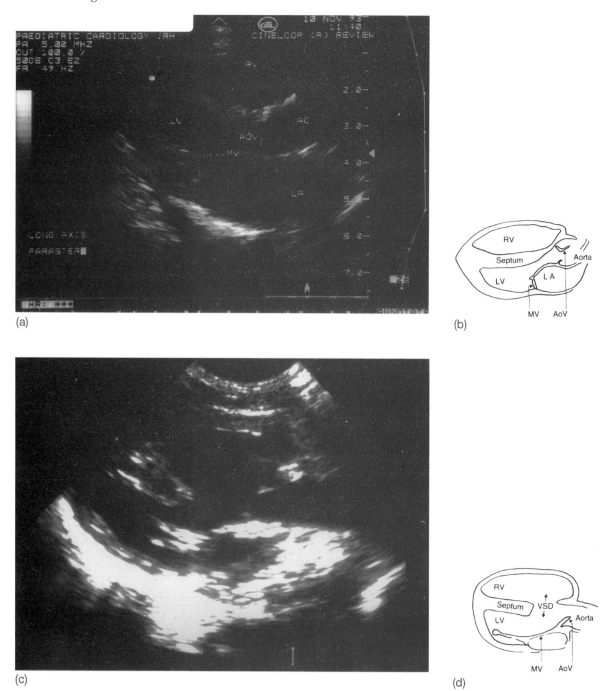

(a)

(b)

(c)

(d)

Figure 2.9   Parasternal long-axis ultrasound scans. (a) Normal heart. (b) Diagram of normal scan. (c) Scan showing outlet VSD, with aorta over-riding the defect so as to arise approximately 50% from each ventricle (in a case of tetralogy of Fallot). (d) Diagram of VSD with aortic over-ride. RV = right ventricle; LV = left ventricle; MV = mitral valve; AoV = aortic valve; LA = left atrium.

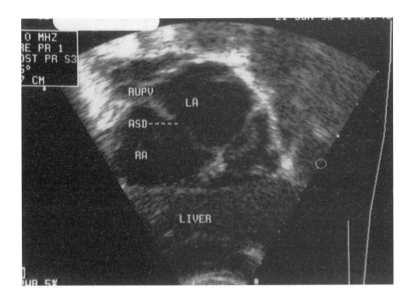

Figure 2.10 Subcostal ultrasound scan. An infant with an ostium secundum ASD. RUPV = right upper pulmonary vein; LA = left atrium; RA = right atrium.

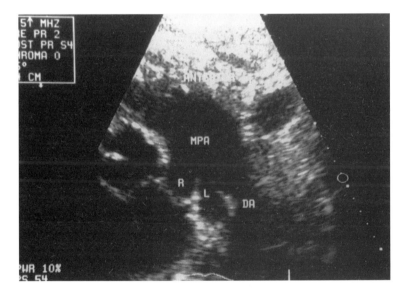

Figure 2.11 Parasternal short-axis ultrasound scan. Large patent ductus arteriosus (DA). MPA = main pulmonary artery; R = right, and L = left pulmonary artery.

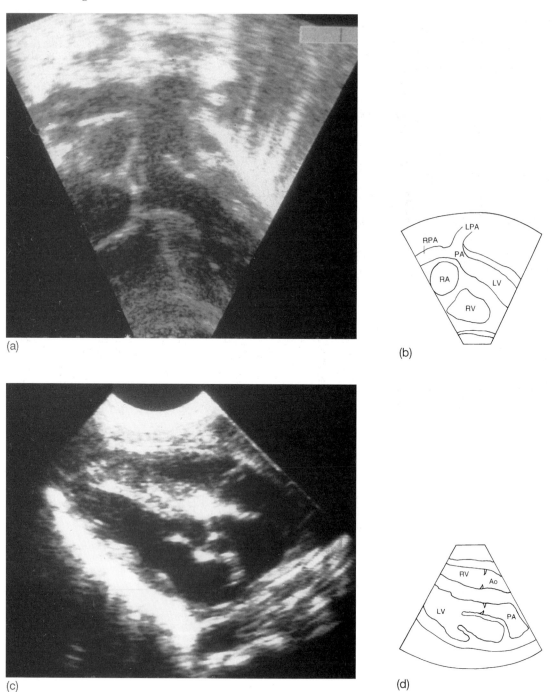

(a)

(b)

(c)

(d)

Figure 2.12   Ultrasound scans showing transposition of the great arteries. (a) Subcostal view showing the pulmonary artery giving rise to right and left branches arising from the left ventricle. (b) Diagram of subcostal view. (c) Parasternal long-axis view showing both great arteries leaving the heart and running parallel rather than crossing over normally. (By kind permission of Dr I. Östman-Smith) (d) Diagram of long-axis view. LPA = left pulmonary artery; RPA = right pulmonary artery; PA = pulmonary artery; Ao = aorta; RA = right atrium; RV = right ventricle; LV = left ventricle.

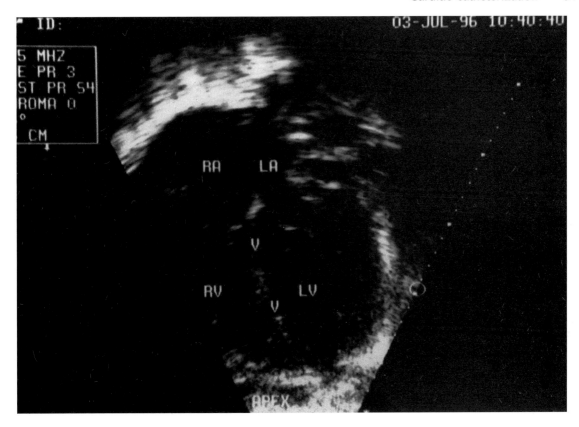

Figure 2.13   Apical four-chamber ultrasound scan. Two muscular VSDs are shown (V).

identifying flow in their respective areas. By convention, red is towards the probe and blue is away from the probe. There is some gradation of colour according to the speed of flow. When all segments display their colour and velocities over a real-time 2D echo, the operator can immediately see the flow characteristics, allowing rapid identification of areas of disturbed flow, e.g. patent ductus, narrow or regurgitant valves, or small ventricular septal defects (VSDs).

Cardiac catheterization

Cardiac catheterization has long been regarded as the gold standard by which other diagnostic imaging techniques are judged. Ultrasound imaging has taken away much of the anatomy-defining role of angiography and Doppler ultrasound allows a great deal of haemodynamic information to be obtained. Angiography is still used to answer specific

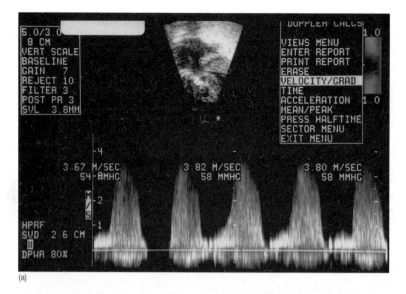

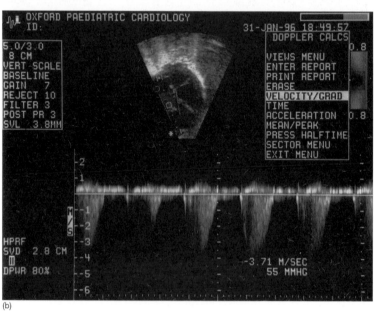

Figure 2.14   Doppler (pulsed wave) traces. (a) High velocity (maximum 3.82 rn/s) signals towards the transducer (displayed as a positive waveform) obtained from a left-to-right shunt through a VSD from the subcostal position. **(b)** Tricuspid regurgitation (away from the transducer) demonstrated from the same position. The jet is also high-velocity, indicating elevated right ventricular pressure.

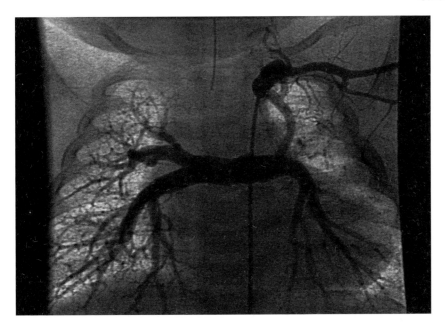

Figure 2.15 Postero-anterior angiogram. Catheter in left subclavian artery; the contrast outlines a surgically created subclavian to pulmonary artery anastomosis (modified Blalock shunt) and the pulmonary vascular tree. The pulmonary arteries are well-grown and not distorted but the left upper lobe supply is not clearly seen. One-year-old child with tetralogy of Fallot and pulmonary atresia.

questions, often in patients who have already had surgical intervention (Figure 2.15).

Haemodynamic data obtained at catheterization is at times crucial to management decisions, particularly in relationship to pulmonary artery pressure and pulmonary vascular resistance. Interventional cardiac catheterization accounts for much of the paediatric use of the catheter laboratory and is considered on pages 51–4.

Depending on the objectives, cardiac catheterization can be performed under sedation and local anaesthesia, and frequently is in infants and adolescents. Toddlers and young children often have general anaesthesia. Vascular access can be obtained *via* the umbilicus in neonates, but most usually at the femoral artery and vein by percutaneous puncture. Other vessels are rarely used and cutdown techniques are seldom necessary.

Morbidity and mortality at diagnostic catheterization was much reduced by the advent of prostaglandin and the availability of ultrasound so that ill newborn babies have a much quicker procedure in a much better condition than previously. Many conditions are now adequately evaluated by ultrasound and proceed directly to palliative or corrective surgery without catheterization. Mortality of paediatric diagnostic cardiac catheterization is less than 1%.

Arterial compromise requiring heparin or streptokinase after the procedure rarely has serious consequences. Serious adverse reactions to contrast medium are rare, as are cerebral embolic phenomena. Infants usually stay in hospital the night after cardiac catheterization but some older children have the procedure as day cases.

Intracardiac electrophysiological studies (EPS) are essentially cardiac catheterizations in which intracardiac electrodes are used to measure time intervals, identify accessory pathways and induce arrhythmias. An EPS provides information of diagnostic value, may result in more rational choice of antiarrhythmic therapy in complex dysrhythmias and is necessary prior to ablation therapy (p. 54).

Magnetic resonance imaging

This technique provides excellent information on cardiac anatomy and has the advantage of involving no radiation exposure. It is particularly useful for imaging the aorta and the pulmonary arteries, but unlike echocardiography it is not a portable investigation and it cannot be combined with interventional techniques, as can angiography at cardiac catheterization. If children require general anaesthesia for MRI there are special precautions with respect to monitoring that need to be taken but even some preschool children can be adequately prepared so that they will lie still for MRI to be performed. The presence of a permanent pacemaker system is a contraindication to MRI but cardiovascular surgical clips and wires are not, even though they may interfere with image quality.

Genetics 3

The incidence of congenital heart disease varies between 5 and 8/1000 live births. There is little variation between nations, although there may be some differences in the type of congenital heart disease involved. For example, the doubly committed ventricular septal defect that leads to fibrous continuity between the aortic and pulmonary valves is commonly seen in Japan, yet is uncommon in other populations. Most surveys of congenital heart disease do not include bicuspid aortic valves, which occur in approximately 1/80 of the population, and other minor abnormalities, e.g. mild pulmonary stenosis and small VSDs, tend to be overlooked. The incidence of varying types of congenital heart disease in the UK is broadly VSD 32%, PDA 12%, pulmonary stenosis 8%, coarctation 6%, ASD 6%, tetralogy of Fallot 6%, aortic stenosis 5%, transposition 5%, hypoplastic left heart 3%, hypoplastic right heart (pulmonary atresia/tricuspid atresia/severe Ebstein's anomaly) 2%, atrioventricular septal defect 2%, truncus arteriosus 1%.

The cause of most cases of congenital heart disease is unknown and is considered to be multifactorial, but it seems the conventional teaching that there is rarely a genetic cause may be wrong. Some genetic causes that are known include chromosomal (gross cytogenetic) defects, single gene lesions (molecular, submicroscopic) and contiguous gene syndromes (subtle cytogenetic or molecular lesions rather than just a single gene defect). Other molecular defects are likely to be documented in the future. In addition some cardiac lesions are linked to teratogens, and maternal disease.

DOWN'S SYNDROME

Chromosomal defects

The best known chromosomal association with congenital heart disease is trisomy 21, or Down's syndrome, which accounts for 5% of all congenital heart disease. The phenotype was first described by John Down in 1866 and the characteristic extra chromosome was identified almost 100 years later. It affects 1/700 live births. Approximately 40% of affected children have congenital heart disease and 40% of these have atrioventricular septal defects (either complete, i.e. with atrial and ventricular defects, or incomplete, with a primum atrioventricular septal defect only). One-third of the 40% with congenital heart disease have ventricular septal defects. Secundum atrial septal defects are seen in 10% and Fallot's tetralogy and patent ductus are both seen in 5% of cases. Other abnormalities are occasionally seen but are uncommon.

Recurrence

The majority of cases of trisomy 21 are caused by non-dysjunction and in 75% of cases this is of maternal origin. The risk is significantly increased with maternal age i.e. 1/1724 at age 20 years, 1/365 at age 35 years, 1/109 at age 40. If a child has a non-dysjunction trisomy 21 the risk of a subsequent affected pregnancy is between 1% and 2%. The recurrence risk is increased if there is translocation or mosaicism in a parent and varies with the site of the translocation or degree of mosaicism. Although most males with Down's syndrome appear to be infertile, there have been a few cases of pregnancy reported in females with Down's syndrome and the recurrence risk of the trisomy has been in the region of 50%.

EDWARDS AND PATAU'S SYNDROMES

Other trisomies associated with congenital heart disease are principally Edwards syndrome (trisomy 18) and Patau's syndrome (trisomy 13). Both are associated with ventricular septal defects, although ASDs and PDAs are also seen quite frequently. Other abnormalities are less common but well recognized, e.g. transposition of the great arteries. Edwards syndrome is typically associated with clenched fists, rocker-bottom feet and micrognathia. Patau's syndrome is often associated with cleft lip and palate, polydactyly and holoprosencephaly. With both of these trisomies the prognosis is extremely poor and cardiac surgery is unwise. Survival is limited by severe neurological problems, which may result in central apnoea, and recurrent seizures.

Trisomies 8 and 9 are rare, but are associated with congenital heart disease. Mosaic trisomies are occasionally seen. An unbalanced translocation involving a trisomy of chromosome 16 is recognized as causing various cardiac abnormalities.

TURNER'S SYNDROME

Turner described this syndrome in 1938. The deficiency of the X chromosome was defined in the 1960s. Only slightly more than half of all cases have typical 45X0; mosaicism and other abnormalities of the X chromosome are common. The incidence is 1/5000–1/10 000 live births, but it is more common antenatally and there is a high spontaneous abortion rate. Most cases are sporadic and the recurrence risk is low. The most consistent of the rather variable features are short stature and gonadal dysgenesis. There is often transient neonatal lymphoedema over the feet and hands. The chest is broad with widely spaced nipples, the ears may be prominent and the mandible small. Neck webbing is seen in approximately half of cases. Cubitus valgus and other skeletal problems may be seen. Renal abnormalities are common (> 60%). Intelligence is normal.

Between 10 and 20% of these girls have cardiac problems which is mainly coarctation of the aorta, although aortic stenosis is also seen. The aortic root can be dilated and dissection is a recognized but uncommon complication whether or not there is coarctation.

Deletions and duplications

Other chromosomal disorders may involve deletions or duplications of part of a chromosome and many are associated with congenital heart disease. They can be detected using banding techniques and it is wise to search for such defects when cardiac disease is found with dysmorphic features, developmental delay, other non-cardiac congenital lesions or a family history. Some of the more common defects that may involve cardiac disease include deletions of 5p (*cri du chat* syndrome), 4p, 4q, 9p, 10q, 13q, 18q and duplications of 3q and 9p. The so called cat-eye syndrome (iris colobomata) is associated with extra material from chromosome 22 and is linked with total anomalous pulmonary venous drainage.

Contiguous gene defects

The distinction between a chromosomal (i.e. gross cytogenetic) defect and a gene (molecular) defect is often difficult, as gene defects are chromosomal, i.e. the locus is on a chromosome. The term 'contiguous gene defect' is used for conditions that are more than 'single' gene defects and DNA or detailed chromosomal analysis can reveal an abnormality. Examples include the following.

BECKWITH–WIEDEMANN SYNDROME

This is caused by duplication of 11p15 and involves hyperplasia and dysplasia of viscera, abdominal wall defects, embryonal cell tumours, cardiac hypertrophy and congenital heart disease.

DIGEORGE ANOMALY

Microdeletion of chromosome 22 within the q11 region is the principal cause of the DiGeorge syndrome (thymic aplasia, hypoparathyroidism and conotruncal cardiac defect) and velocardiofacial/shprintzen syndrome (palatal abnormalities, heart defects and dysmorphic facial features). It is now recognized that there is a spectrum of disease associated with this chromosomal problem and the acronym CATCH 22 syndrome is used to encompass this – C = cardiac; A = abnormal facies; T = thymic hypoplasia; C = cleft palate; H = hypocalcaemia.

It has been suggested that the features can be divided into the common (facial features, developmental delay), common but not universal (conotruncal cardiac lesion, thymic aplasia) and rare (upper limb abnormality, meningomyelocele, cerebellar atrophy and probably renal abnormalities, although these may be more common than initially realized). The rarer lesions have been postulated to be related to a genetic 'second hit'.

There is variability of phenotypic expression among familial cases (and therefore presumably identical deletions). The facial features probably represent abnormal development of the mesenchymal structures of the face. The nose is often prominent, palpebral fissures are narrow, there is a long face and a small chin. The cleft of the palate is either overt or submucous. Speech is usually nasal and often delayed. Learning disabilities tend to be mild rather than severe, with IQs usually above 50 but less than 100.

The true prevalence of the genetic abnormality is uncertain, as most cases are diagnosed after a cardiac lesion has been detected. The incidence has been estimated at 1/10 000 but may be 1/4000 or higher if mild cases (without cardiac abnormalities) are included. The DiGeorge anomaly may cause approximately 5% of congenital heart disease. A significant number of familial cases have been recognized and most carrier parents are asymptomatic (Figure 3.1). Monozygotic twins with the deletion but with different cardiac defects have been described. Diagnosis is now quite rapid, using fluorescence *in situ* hybridization (FISH).

The cardiac lesions are described as 'conotruncal' as they typically involve outflow tracts (conus) of the heart. The most frequent lesions are truncus arteriosus, interrupted aortic arch and Fallot's tetralogy with pulmonary atresia. The more usual Fallot's tetralogy without pulmonary atresia is rarely associated with this chromosome defect, although some do advocate screening in all cases of tetralogy. Other less commonly associated lesions include ventricular septal defect, absent pulmonary valve syndrome, anomalous origin of the pulmonary artery from the aorta (hemitruncus), right aortic arch, vascular ring and coarctation. A deletion in 22q11 should be considered when there is

Plates

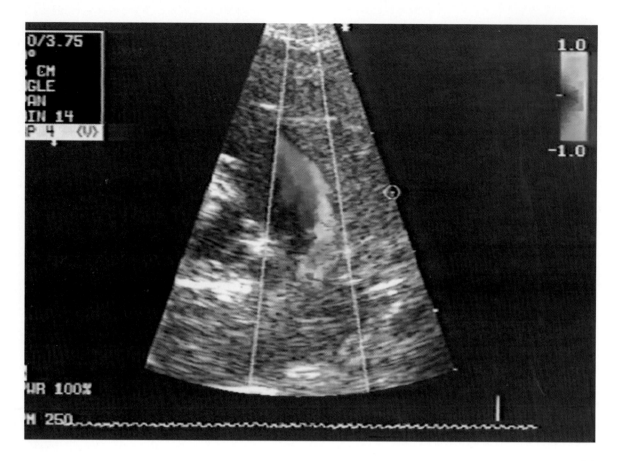

(a)

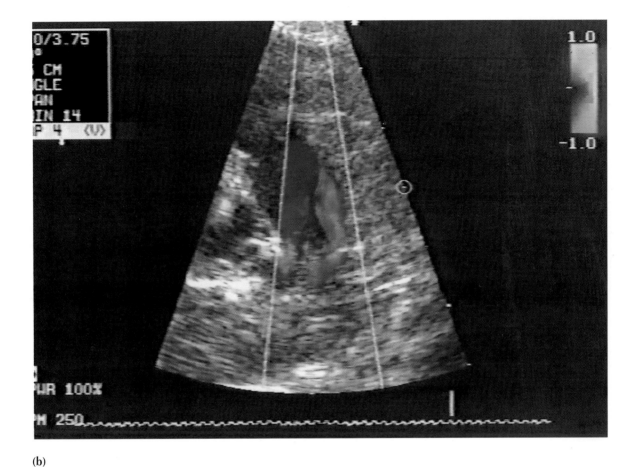

(b)

Plate 1 **(a, b) Colour flow Doppler ultrasound**. Two parasternal long-axis views demonstrating left-to-right shunting through a patent ductus arteriosus. In each case left-to-right shunting is towards the transducer and is therefore displayed as a predominantly red signal; forward flow in the pulmonary artery towards the lungs is away from the transducer and is displayed in blue.

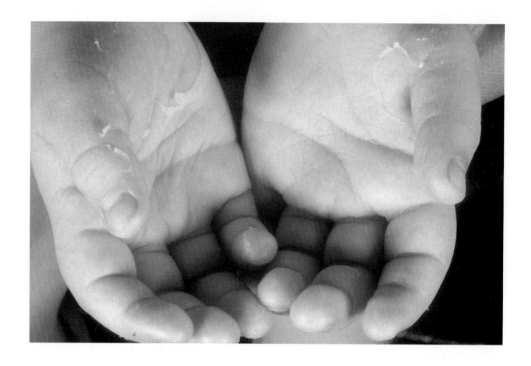

Plate 2　Peeling hands in the convalescent phase of Kawasaki's disease. By kind permission of Dr I. Östman-Smith.

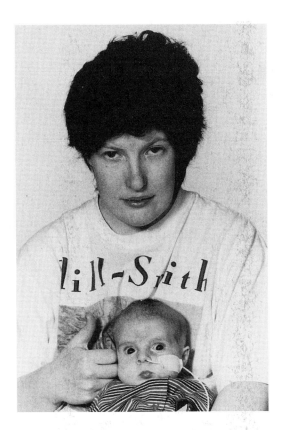

Figure 3.1   22q11 deletion. A mother and young infant, both of whom have 22q11 deletion. The mother has a normal heart; the infant has truncus arteriosus (repaired). Reproduced by kind permission of the mother.

family history of congenital heart disease or dysmorphic features with heart disease, or if thymic aplasia is found at cardiac surgery.

The immune deficiency associated with thymic aplasia should lead to precautions when the diagnosis is suspected. Blood products should be irradiated to prevent graft *versus* host disease and live vaccines such as BCG should be avoided until a detailed immunological assessment has been made. Often there is a tendency to frequent respiratory infections, although this tends to improve with age. Approximately 20–30% of cases of truncus arteriosus or interrupted aortic arch are associated with 22q11 deletions and when emergency surgery is considered in these cases, prior to chromosome and T cell analysis, blood products should always be irradiated to prevent graft *versus* host disease. The hypo-calcaemia associated with DiGeorge syndrome seems to be most severe in the neonatal period and improves in childhood. Once the chromosomal diagnosis is established it is important to undertake a full survey for immunodeficiency and hypocalcaemia, and the palate should be examined. The possibility of velopharyngeal insufficiency and developmental delay should be considered with appropriate early involvement of allied specialties. Late psychiatric problems have been documented in 22q11 deficiency and should be considered in long-term follow-up of these cases.

WILLIAMS SYNDROME

Sporadic Williams syndrome, and inherited cases of supravalvar aortic stenosis without the other features, are now recognized to be due to gene deletion syndromes within the elastin gene locus on chromosome 7. There may be contiguous genes in the microdeletions that account for the varied abnormalities in the syndrome. A FISH screen is available, which offers rapid diagnosis of the abnormality. Williams first described this problem in 1961. The facial features are typical (Figure

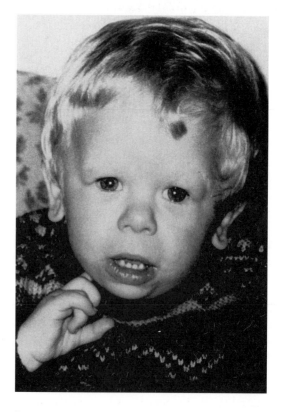

Figure 3.2   Williams syndrome in an 18-month-old child. Reproduced by kind permission of the family.

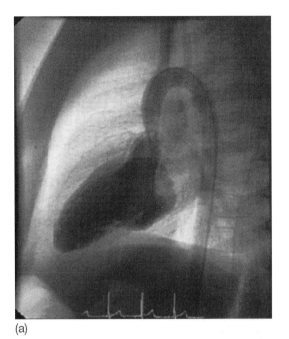
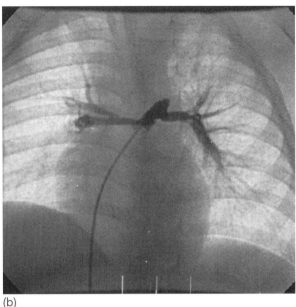

(a)   (b)

Figure 3.3 (a) **Left ventricular angiogram**. Lateral projection, showing supravalvar aortic narrowing (catheter entering the heart *via* the femoral artery and the aorta) (b) **Pulmonary angiogram**. Antero-posterior view, showing multiple pulmonary artery branch stenoses, which cause sudden reductions in vessel calibre at bifurcations rather than normal smooth progressive changes (patient with Williams syndrome).

3.2), but often develop during childhood, the features being difficult to diagnose in infancy but more obvious in older children and adults.

The average IQ is around 50 and the personality has been described as 'cocktail party': in general affected individuals tend to be outgoing, loquacious and friendly. The facial features include broad lips and nose with anteverted nares and a long philtrum. There is often a prominent periorbital fullness and a depressed nasal bridge. Palpable fissures are usually short. A typical stellate pattern is seen in the iris.

The cardiac lesions principally consist of supravalvular aortic stenosis with a typically flask-shaped aortic root, enlarged aortic sinuses and a narrow ascending aorta (Figure 3.3(a)). The supravalvular aortic stenosis tends to be progressive. There is often peripheral pulmonary artery stenosis (Figure 3.3(b)), which can be quite severe but often improves over time.

Aortic and pulmonary valve stenoses are occasionally seen, as are septal defects and coarctation of the aorta. The aorta can be quite hypoplastic and sometimes renal artery stenoses are found, which can cause hypertension. Other arterial anomalies are sometimes found with stenotic areas or hypoplasia. Occasionally cardiac surgery is needed for supravalvar aortic stenosis and can involve extensive reconstruction of the aortic root. In families with isolated cardiac involvement the condition behaves as a single gene (rather than contiguous gene) disorder.

Feeding difficulties are very well recognized in babies and they are often fretful. Hypercalcaemia may be seen in infancy but tends to improve with time; it can be intermittent.

MILLER–DIEKER SYNDROME

This is caused by deletion of 17p13 and involves lissencephaly, i.e. a smooth brain surface, a furrow in the central forehead, a dysmorphic face and congenital heart disease.

Single gene diseases associated with congenital heart disease

AUTOSOMAL DOMINANT

Noonan's syndrome

Noonan's syndrome (described by Noonan in 1963) consists of short stature, cardiac lesions and typical facial features (Figure 3.4).

The latter include hypertelorism and low-set, posteriorly rotated ears. Ptosis and squint are common. The posterior hairline is low and the neck is sometimes webbed. In boys cryptorchidism is very common. Skeletal, renal and clotting abnormalities are sometimes seen. The hair is often curly and multiple pigmented lesions are quite common. The skeletal abnormalities include a typically abnormal chest shape with pectus excavatum/carinatum. Noonan's syndrome has recently been mapped in one large family to an area of chromosome 12, but there does appear to be genetic heterogeneity. There is clear overlap with leopard syndrome, an acronym for: L = lentigines; E = ECG abnormalities; O = ocular hypertelorism; P = pulmonary stenosis; A = abnormalities of the genitalia; R = retardation of growth; D = deafness. Many people now consider that leopard and Noonan's syndromes are part of the same spectrum. The ECG with leopard syndrome tends to show prolongation of the PR interval and abnormal P waves, whereas with Noonan's syndrome the QRS axis tends to be superior. Both syndromes are associated with hypertrophic cardiomyopathy and pulmonary stenosis. Other abnormalities of leopard syndrome are all found with Noonan's syndrome, including deafness. Both demonstrate autosomal dominant inheritance.

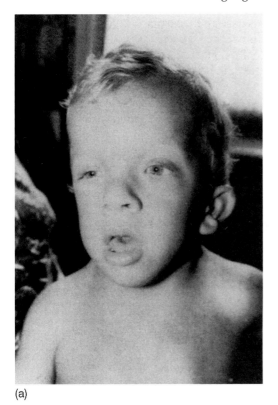
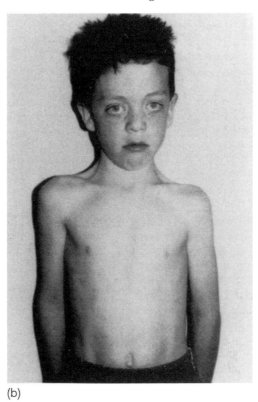

(a)   (b)

Figure 3.4 Noonan's syndrome (a) in a toddler and (b) in a 5 year old boy. Reproduced by kind permission of the families; from Sharland *et al.*, *Arch Dis Child* 1992; 67: 178–183, with permission of BMJ Publishing Group.

Developmental delay and specific learning problems are common but not universal in Noonan's syndrome; severe mental retardation is uncommon and should lead to consideration of another diagnosis. Most cases of Noonan's syndrome are sporadic. Antenatally, a cardiac lesion may be seen or there may be polyhydramnios; cystic hygroma formation is sometimes seen. Postnatally, feeding difficulties are common and gastro-oesophageal reflux may be severe.

The pulmonary stenosis associated with Noonan's syndrome is often difficult to treat with balloon valvuloplasty as the valve is commonly dysplastic, i.e. thickened and immobile. Cardiac surgery is often required. Hypertrophic cardiomyopathy is present to a varying degree in around 20% of cases of Noonan's syndrome. With severe cases there can be heart failure and death in infancy. Less severe cases can survive to childhood. Occasionally, the physiology is more restrictive rather than hypertrophic. Secundum atrial septal defects are seen not infrequently, but other abnormalities are much less common.

Marfan's syndrome

Marfan first described the phenotype in 1896. Typically there is tall stature (above and proceeding parallel to the 97th centile) with long fingers, increased span and reduced upper-to-lower-body ratio. Joints are lax and scoliosis/kyphoscoliosis and pectus are common. The palate is high and arched and retrognathia is also frequent. Myopia is often severe and is seen in over 50% of cases. Lens dislocation is well recognized. Retinal detachments may occur. Inguinal hernias and pneumothoraces are other known complications. Spinal root irritation can occur because of dural ectasia causing protrusion.

There appears to be a deficiency of fibrillin (a ubiquitous glycoprotein) in Marfan's patients, caused by various mutations of the fibrillin gene (on chromosome 15q), although other fibrillin-like genes seem to be responsible for some cases.

The typical cardiac finding with Marfan's syndrome is echocardiographic evidence of aortic root dilatation and as this progressively enlarges there is an increased tendency to aortic dissection. The latter is uncommon in childhood, being more common when the aortic root measures over 5 cm. It can result in sudden death. The pain of dissection is typically very severe and is described as tearing, radiating to the back or neck. The extent of the dissection (which is usually progressive distally, although occasionally the aorta may dissect to the coronaries) is assessed with transoesophageal echo or with MRI. Sometimes CT or angiography are used. Elective aortic root replacement is now advocated when the dilatation is over 5.5 cm but with improved surgical technique this is now being done earlier. Mitral valve prolapse is frequently seen in both children and adults and can lead to progressive mitral regurgitation. Aortic regurgitation too is frequently found and is progressive as the aortic root dilates.

Beta-blocker therapy is felt to reduce the risk of dissection and is often used in children with Marfan's syndrome, particularly if there is a family history of dissection, as this significantly increases the risk. Strenuous exercise and contact sports should be avoided as they could precipitate a dissection. Blood pressure should be monitored regularly as hypertension leads to an increased risk. Echocardiography is performed regularly and a rapid increase in aortic root size, or an absolute measurement above the level considered unsafe to leave (this varies among cardiac centres as discussed above), should lead to surgical referral. Recent studies suggest that life expectancy with Marfan's syndrome has improved. This is probably because of the widespread use of beta-blockers and improved surgical techniques for elective and acute aortic root surgery. The average life expectancy is around 40–50 years, slightly better for women than men.

Holt–Oram syndrome

Holt and Oram described this condition in 1960. The typical cardiac lesion with Holt–Oram syndrome is the secundum atrial septal defect and it is associated with an upper limb abnormality. Inheritance is autosomal dominant. Occasionally, ventricular septal defects are seen and rarely other cardiac problems. The upper limb is exclusively involved, often asymmetrically with the radial ray predominantly affected. The severity varies between minor clinodactyly and severe reduction deformities, and there appears to be increasing severity with succeeding generations. Although Holt–Oram syndrome appears to be genetically heterogeneous one locus has been mapped to the region of chromosome 12q2.

Other dominant lesions

Other autosomal dominant lesions include familial atrial septal defects (although most ASDs are not familial) and familial total anomalous pulmonary venous drainage (which appears to have a low penetrance); the latter has been linked to chromosome 4. Patent ductus is sometimes familial with dominant, recessive and multifactorial inheritance all reported. Hypertrophic cardiomyopathy is inherited as an autosomal dominant trait; this is discussed in Chapter 11.

Another syndrome with autosomal dominant inheritance and cardiac disease is Apert's syndrome. The cardiac lesion is pulmonary stenosis and/or ventricular septal defect. There is craniosynostosis with syndactyly and deafness.

Myotonic dystrophy is also dominant. The most common lesion is a conduction defect seen on the ECG. In addition to characteristic myotonia there may be typical facial features, ptosis, cataracts and frontal balding.

There may also be a number of new mutations of autosomal dominant genes that were previously concealed by the high mortality from the cardiac lesions but, as surgery for complex congenital heart disease improves, a number of young people are surviving to reproduce and some conditions appear to have an increased recurrence in offspring, suggesting a possibly dominant inheritance.

AUTOSOMAL RECESSIVE

The following conditions exhibit recessive inheritance.

- **Carpenter's syndrome**: craniosynostosis, polydactyly and varied cardiac lesions (including septal defects, pulmonary stenosis and patent ductus).
- **Ellis–van Creveld syndrome**: polydactyly, short limbs, sparse hair, abnormal teeth and nails, and cardiac disease (septal defects) in 50%.
- **Homocystinuria** is due to cystathionine synthase deficiency. There is a Marfanoid appearance but lens dislocation tends to be downwards and inwards as opposed to the upwards and outwards dislocation of Marfan's syndrome. There is an increased tendency to vascular thrombosis.
- **Kartagener's syndrome**: the cardiac lesion is dextrocardia, although the heart is structurally normal in most cases. In addition to dextrocardia there is mirror image situs inversus and usually ciliary dyskinesis with a tendency to recurrent chest infection and ultimately bronchiectasis.
- **Pompe's disease** is discussed in Chapter 11.
- **Isomerism**: the isomerism complex appears recessively inherited in some families. In essence the syndrome involves duplication of left- or right-sided structures. With left isomerism both atria have a left atrial morphology, as do both lungs, there is polysplenia and the azygous vein connects to the superior vena cava (the inferior vena cava does not drain to the heart). There can be dextrocardia. While these abnormalities may not cause any problems there is an increased incidence of congenital heart disease. The severity of congenital heart disease is greater when there is right isomerism (both atria and lungs having a right-sided appearance) and total anomalous pulmonary venous drainage; atrioventricular septal defect, double-outlet right ventricle and pulmonary atresia can be seen together, often with dextrocardia. After initial complex palliation these children will require a total cavopulmonary (Fontan-type) connection. Many will not survive surgery and additional morbidity and mortality are recognized as a result of the associated asplenia, which requires lifelong prophylaxis with oral penicillin.
- **Ehlers–Danlos syndrome**: both recessive and dominant forms have been described. There is hyperextensibility of the skin, which is thin and bruises easily. The cardiac lesions include aortic dissection and aneurysm, atrial septal defects and mitral valve prolapse.

OTHERS

The increased incidence of congenital heart disease in consanguineous families suggests that some isolated heart defects may be recessively inherited; for example, some cases of hypoplastic left heart, pulmonary atresia and Ebstein's anomaly exhibit recessive inheritance patterns.

Duchenne muscular dystrophy is X-linked and is associated with a cardiomyopathy. A form of dilated cardiomyopathy has (like Duchenne dystrophy) been mapped to the dystrophin gene, but there is no associated skeletal myopathy. Some other forms of congenital heart disease have also been suggested to have X-linked transmission, including dextrocardia with structural heart disease and left-sided valve disease.

X-linked inheritance

Table 3.1 lists known teratogens for congenital heart disease.

Teratogens

Table 3.1   Known teratogens for congenital heart disease

Teratogen	*Most frequent cardiac malformation*
Alcohol (in high doses), amphetamines and cocaine	Septal defects and/or transposition
Phenytoin	Aortic and pulmonary stenosis, coarctation, PDA
Warfarin	Various defects
Lithium	Ebstein's anomaly
Carbamazepine	ASD, PDA
Trimethodione (an anticonvulsant)	Transposition/tetralogy
Sodium valproate	Tetralogy of Fallot, ventricular septal defect
Thalidomide (now never used in pregnancy)	Tetralogy, septal defects
Methotrexate, cyclophosphamide, daunorubicin	Tetralogy, dextrocardia
Viruses (principally rubella)	PDA, peripheral pulmonary stenosis, septal defects

The following maternal diseases are linked with an increased risk of congenital heart disease:

Maternal disease

- **diabetes**: transposition, septal defects, coarctation, ventricular hypertrophy;

- **phenylketonuria**: tetralogy of Fallot;
- **systemic lupus erythematosus**: complete heart block.

Twin studies have shown an increased incidence of congenital heart disease in monozygotic twins, perhaps as much as twice the normal rate. This may be related to the twinning process itself. It does appear that twin-to-twin transfusion with changes in right ventricular loading conditions can lead to right-sided heart disease, including pulmonary atresia.

Recurrence of congenital heart disease

As discussed above, some cases of congenital heart disease can be linked to a chromosomal defect, a single gene disorder or a teratogen, but in approximately 80% of cases the cause of congenital heart disease is unknown. In these cases the recurrence risk in the offspring of affected probands is generally greater than in siblings. The risk of congenital heart disease in subsequent pregnancies when one child has been affected is in the region of 1/50. The figure increases to 1/10 if a second child is affected. The recurrence risk for specific congenital heart disease varies from between 1% and 3% once single gene inheritance is excluded. The risk in the offspring of affected parents is commonly 5%, although this is less with the isomerism sequence, which may be recessive.

Other syndromes

In addition to Mendelian inheritance there are many syndromes that are associated with congenital heart disease but are sporadic. However, they may be linked to contiguous genes or single gene lesions in the future. These include the following.

- **Alagille's syndrome** is the association of chronic cholestasis with cardiac disease, which is typically peripheral pulmonary stenosis but occasionally may be cyanotic heart disease such as tetralogy of Fallot. Approximately one-third of cases have skeletal abnormalities. There are abnormal facies and a posterior embryotoxon (on slit-lamp examination) in the majority of cases. Skeletal, renal, neural and endocrine problems have been described. Arteriovenous malformations may develop in the lung probably secondary to chronic hepatic dysfunction. It is possible that inheritance may be autosomal dominant with reduced penetrance and there is linkage to chromosome 20p11.2.
- **Pentalogy of Cantrell.** The typical cardiac lesion is tetralogy of Fallot and in addition there is a defect of the chest and abdominal wall with a bifid or short sternum, gastroschisis and absent diaphragm.

- **Charge syndrome** is an acronym that represents: C = colobomata of the iris and/or the retina; H = heart defect (a wide variety, including both ventricular and atrioventricular septal defects, tetralogy of Fallot and double-outlet right ventricle); A = atresia of the choanae; R = retardation (this is principally of growth, although most children are developmentally delayed – a few cases may have normal intelligence); G = genitalia (the genitalia is small in boys); E = ear deformity, which is varied but can be a large, floppy or cup-shaped ear and there is often associated deafness.
- **De Lange's syndrome.** The cardiac lesions are usually septal defects. Other abnormalities include severe mental retardation, abnormally bushy eyebrows, hirsutism, microcephaly and short stature.
- **Goldenhar syndrome.** A variety of cardiac lesions are reported, including ventricular septal defects and Fallot's tetralogy. Other problems include epibulbar dermoid, preauricular skin tags, colobomata, cleft palate, vertebral anomalies and hemifacial microsomia.
- **Kabuki make-up syndrome.** A variety of heart defects are associated, including ventricular septal defect and double-outlet right ventricle. The face is characteristic, with tented eyebrows and abnormal lips, eyes and ears.
- **Klippel–Feil syndrome.** Septal defects are most commonly seen with this syndrome, which has a characteristic short neck.
- **VACTERL** is an acronym for: V = vertebral anomalies; A = anal atresia; C = cardiac defect; T = tracheal-oesophageal fistula; R = renal anomalies; L = limb defects. The cardiac lesions are varied but are most commonly ventricular septal defects or tetralogy of Fallot.
- **Rubinstein–Taybi syndrome.** VSDs or PDAs are seen in approximately one-third of patients. Broad thumbs (and sometimes fingers and toes), short stature, facial dysmorphism and an IQ of less than 100 (often < 60) are other features.

Interventions 4

In this chapter brief consideration will be given to interventional cardiac catheterization and surgery. Any intervention aimed at altering haemodynamics can be viewed as either palliative or corrective. Corrective procedures can be further classified as either anatomically corrective, as in obliterating a shunt lesion, or physiologically corrective, as in separating oxygenated and deoxygenated blood. An example of a physiologically corrective procedure would be the Fontan operation for tricuspid atresia, in which the right atrium is attached to the pulmonary artery, thereby diverting systemic venous drainage directly into the lungs and returning systemic arterial saturation to normal without returning cardiovascular anatomy to normal. The question remains as to whether or not an anatomical correction restores complete normality and can then be regarded as a cure. For example, an operation may not reduce the risk of endocarditis to that of the population as a whole or may be associated with long-term increased susceptibility to rhythm disturbances. There are only a few procedures for which these criteria of complete cure can be claimed with confidence, such as total occlusion of a patent ductus arteriosus.

Interventional cardiac catheterization

Vascular access is discussed in Chapter 2. Procedures are usually done under general anaesthesia or at least under very heavy sedation.

BALLOON SEPTOSTOMY

Balloon septostomy was pioneered by Rashkind for transposition and involves passing a balloon catheter through the foramen ovale into the left atrium. The balloon is then inflated and the catheter is given a short, hard jerk back into the right atrium, thereby tearing and enlarging the foramen ovale. In transposition this will usually improve oxygenation by increasing mixing of blood sufficient to prevent or reverse metabolic acidosis. It needs to be performed urgently in transposition of the great arteries if improving ductal patency with prostaglandin does not adequately increase oxygenation or if early arterial switch operation is not intended. Balloon septostomy can be carried out with low morbidity and mortality under ultrasound control rather than X-ray screening and therefore does not necessarily need transfer of the infant from the neonatal unit to the cardiac catheter laboratory. Enlargement of the foramen ovale by balloon septostomy may also be indicated when exit of blood from either atrium through tricuspid or mitral valves is seriously impaired, for example in mitral atresia with double-outlet right ventricle, or pulmonary atresia and a small tricuspid valve.

BALLOON DILATATION

This is increasingly used as an alternative to surgery for a range of conditions (Table 4.1) and the excellence of results obtained for pulmonary valve stenosis and recoarctation make it the procedure of choice for these conditions.

Procedures outside the newborn period have a low morbidity and mortality. In the newborn period the choice between balloon dilatation and surgery will vary from centre to centre.

OCCLUSION OF SHUNTS

Occlusion of the ductus arteriosus by umbrella devices or more recently by coils (Figure 4.1) is widely carried out but is not yet suitable for premature infants.

Surgical clipping or ligation of the ductus has a somewhat higher success rate for complete occlusion but repeat interventional catheterization can be performed if a less than satisfactory result is obtained at the first attempt. Surgery does involve a longer hospital stay. Radiation exposure occurs with umbrella or coil occlusion. Surgery is associated with postoperative discomfort and a scar, but catheter occlusion can result in important venous or arterial damage. Catheter-delivered device closure of secundum atrial septal defects has been introduced in many centres; the various devices are being evaluated. Not all defects are suitable and medium- and long-term results are unknown. Embolization of systemic-to-pulmonary collaterals and of both pulmonary and systemic arteriovenous fistulae is often the treatment of choice.

STENTING

Indwelling intravascular stents are used as a primary procedure or after balloon dilatation in pulmonary arterial stenoses, mainly those seen in older children and young adults with complicated tetralogy of Fallot

Table 4.1 Interventional cardiac catheterization (1 = catheter therapy treatment of choice; 2 = catheter therapy commonly used, though surgery widely used also; 3 = surgery generally preferable but catheter treatment may be indicated in certain circumstances; 4 = surgery preferable; 5 = catheter intervention being evaluated in many centres)

Lesion	Catheter treatment	Comments
Pulmonary valve stenosis	1	
Stenosed venous pathways post-Mustard/Senning operations	1	
AV malformations	1	
Re-coarctation	1	
Critical pulmonary stenosis, neonatal	2	
Aortic stenosis	2	
Neonatal critical aortic stenosis	2	
Pulmonary artery branch stenosis	2	Balloon followed by stenting
Patient ductus arteriosus, later infancy onwards	2	
Native coarctation	3	
Pulmonary atresia with intact ventricular septum	3	Laser perforation of valve followed by balloon
Tetralogy of Fallot	3	Balloon can palliate instead of a surgical systemic-to-pulmonary anastomosis
Ventricular septal defect	3	
Stenosed surgical systemic-to-pulmonary anastomosis	3	
Patent ductus arteriosus, preterm infant	4	
Aortic atresia	4	
Atrial septal defect	5	

and similar lesions. In many of these patients surgery has previously failed to give lasting relief of obstruction or may even have precipitated distortion and stenosis. Stenosed venous pathways after intra-atrial surgery for transposition (Mustard and Senning operations) can be dilated and stented, and major aorto-pulmonary collateral arteries can be either blocked with a coil or stented open depending on whether

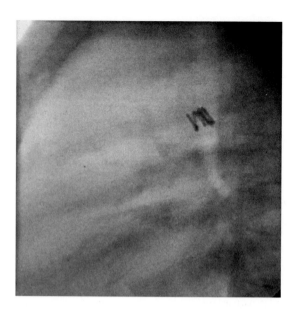

Figure 4.1   Lateral chest X-ray. Screening picture during cardiac catheterization showing a coil placed in the ductus arteriosus to occlude it.

there is too much or to little pulmonary blood flow. Stenting the ductus arteriosus is being explored as part of the palliation of hypoplastic left heart syndrome, in conjunction with pulmonary artery branch banding, although the Norwood operation appears to be the most widely adopted initial palliation (p. 187).

ABLATION

Removal of foci of arrhythmias and interruption of accessory pathways are now done by catheter ablation using radiofrequency. Such intervention is rarely needed in young children but the attraction of abolishing arrhythmias by ablation and removing the need for long-term medication is considerable in older children and adolescents. Many arrhythmias in younger children are ultimately self limiting and the technique of catheter ablation is much easier in larger children. See Chapter 14 for detailed consideration of arrhythmia therapy and indications for catheter ablation.

Conventional surgery   Cardiac surgical procedures are described as either closed or open and may be performed through a lateral thoracotomy (usually closed operations) or from the front, most commonly through a median sternotomy incision (Table 4.2).

Table 4.2 Types of cardiovascular surgery

	Usual incision
Closed operations	
Patent ductus arteriosus	Lateral thoracotomy
Coarctation	
Systemic-to-pulmonary anastomosis (Blalock type shunt)	
Pulmonary artery banding	
Central systemic-to-pulmonary anastomosis (ascending aorta to pulmonary artery)	Median sternotomy
Open heart operations	
Intracardiac procedures	Median sternotomy

The sternum is often repaired with radio-opaque wire. Temporary pacing wires are usually removed a few days postoperatively but are occasionally cut at the skin, in which case they will be detectable on X-ray thereafter. Blood vessels are often occluded with metal clips, which are radio-opaque. Wires and clips are not a contraindication to magnetic resonance imaging, although they may interfere with image quality. Thoracoscopic clipping of the ductus arteriosus has been investigated in some centres.

Open heart surgery requires the heart to be stopped, which is achieved with a cold electrolyte solution (cardioplegia solution). Permanent damage to vital organs is prevented either by the use of deep hypothermia or by circulation being maintained by cardiopulmonary bypass. Both techniques can be used in the same operation, bypass being used to achieve cooling and rewarming while some of the repair itself is done without bypass being employed.

In general the longer the time on bypass and the longer the period of hypothermic arrest the more cerebral, pulmonary and renal dysfunction is likely to occur in the first few postoperative days. Postoperative intensive care may involve not only cardiac support but also ventilation and dialysis. In the region of 15–20% of infants have been reported to have fits within 72 hours of open heart surgery; in the majority these do not persist and are not an indicator for long-term cerebral sequelae.

Cardiac surgery may occasionally damage the recurrent laryngeal nerve, which can cause variable upper airway problems in the early postoperative period and can result in a weak or hoarse cry. Usually, the problem resolves spontaneously although occasionally the damage is permanent. The phrenic nerve can also be damaged surgically. Similarly, this problem usually resolves spontaneously over 3–6 months although it is occasionally permanent. In older children this does not cause significant respiratory difficulties, but in infancy it can cause quite marked ventilator dependence. Plication of the diaphragm is sometimes required to wean the child successfully. The diagnosis is usually established with ultrasound screening. The paralysed diaphragm is seen to move paradoxically on the affected side (i.e. cephalad with inspiration).

Chylothorax can complicate cardiothoracic surgery. Although this tends to resolve spontaneously, a low-fat, medium chain triglyceride diet is often used to try to reduce the volume of chyle. Total parenteral nutrition has been used in these circumstances and sometimes pleurodesis is required. Excessive chyle loss can cause hypoalbuminaemia and compromise immune function because of the loss of lymphocytes. Children left with high systemic venous pressures may be prone to recurrent or chronic pleural effusions and even ascites and troublesome peripheral oedema. These occurrences are particularly associated with Fontan-type circulations where the systemic veins are connected directly to the pulmonary arterial tree, and a few such patients can also develop malabsorption, with protein-losing enteropathy related to high venous pressures in the intestinal tract. Cervical sympathetic dysfunction (Horner's syndrome) is a common and usually transient occurrence after coarctation repair and Blalock-type systemic to pulmonary arterial anastomoses.

Pericardial effusions (Figure 4.2) can occur acutely postoperatively or some weeks or months later, in which case they are likely to be manifestations of the post-pericardotomy syndrome (see page 118). Tamponade can occur in the early postoperative period or later in association with the post-pericardotomy syndrome; its onset can be rapid and may require urgent aspiration or drainage.

Before discharge from hospital infants and children have to be seen to be haemodynamically stable on the right doses of medication and in the case of small babies having an acceptable feeding regime. All families should be given clear written advice about postoperative care at home and discharge advice to family doctors and local paediatricians must highlight specific problem areas. Particular points to be covered for families and professionals are listed in Table 4.3.

Transplantation   The commonest cause for heart transplantation in children is dilated cardiomyopathy, but increasingly children with congenital heart disease are being transplanted and it is quite possible that the latter may become the commonest cause for transplantation in the future. The short-term results of transplantation are reasonably good, with a high survival for the first 2 years (80% or more). The initial attrition is often perioperative and is related to acute failure of the transplanted organ. There may be a problem because of poor preservation of the myocardium, hyperacute rejection or an underestimation of the pulmonary vascular resistance such that the new right ventricle cannot cope with

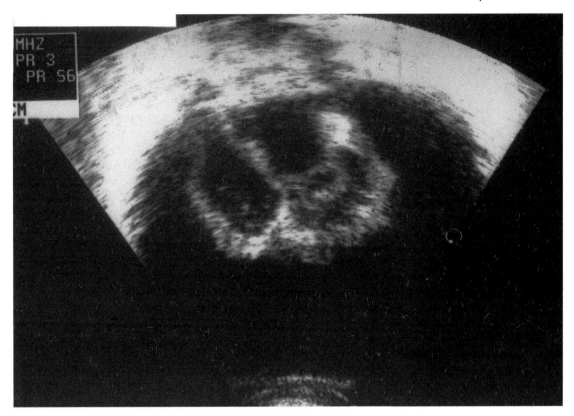

Figure 4.2 Subcostal ultrasound scan. The heart is surrounded by a very large pericardial effusion (in a case of post-pericardotomy syndrome).

the work required. In the early post-transplant period heavy immunosuppression is given and severe infections may occur. In the medium term deaths can occur from infection or high-grade rejection, but increasingly cardiologists are seeing children with coronary artery problems which are probably related to chronic low-grade rejection. These can be severe enough to cause a sudden death or chronic heart failure. Retransplantation is sometimes undertaken, but the coronary changes may reoccur, sometimes more rapidly. In addition, there is an increased incidence of lymphomas and other malignancies because of the immunosuppression schedule. Growth is often suppressed because of steroid therapy and cyclosporin may cause chronic hypertension as well as unsightly hirsutism.

Heart–lung transplantation is also undertaken in children, e.g. in cystic fibrosis or pulmonary hypertension. The results of heart–lung transplantation are worse than those of heart transplantation. It seems

Table 4.3 Advice about postoperative care for families of cardiac surgery patients

Topic	Comments
Wound care	Keep dry until scabs fall off
	Seek help if red/swollen/discharge
School	Return 2 weeks after leaving hospital
Exercise	No need to restrict exertion **but** no contact sports for 3 months (make relevant to age)
Medication	Many are on diuretics after open heart surgery, aspirin after systemic to pulmonary anastomoses and antihypertensives after coarctation repair; ensure that the need for repeat prescriptions is understood
Endocarditis	Remind about prevention (applies to all postoperative cases, although only for 3 months for completely occluded PDA and straightforward secundum ASD)
Behaviour	Post-surgery and post-hospital emotional lability, some temporary regression in younger children (bed-wetting, sleep disturbance, feeding difficulties)
Post-pericardotomy syndrome	Medical help to be sought if fever, cough, breathlessness or flu-like symptoms occur (p. 118–19)

that the majority of children develop an obliterative bronchiolitis, which may be due to chronic rejection.

Paediatricians are often asked to share care of transplanted patients. This will involve checking cyclosporin levels and monitoring azathioprine dose by assessing the suppression of the white cell count. Sometimes ECGs and echocardiograms are undertaken locally to avoid frequent travel to a cardiac centre. Patients will often seek advice about contact with infectious diseases; in general the same rules apply as to other patients with a suppressed immune system. Immune status to common childhood illnesses is checked as part of the transplant assessment. After transplant contact with a child with an illness to which the child is not immune should be treated appropriately. Live vaccinations should be avoided. In general it is advised to be cautious over contact with others in the first few months after transplant as the immunosuppression is greater, but later on the children should be able to return to normal schooling and activities.

Heart and heart–lung transplantation (and recently single lung transplantation) are pioneering surgical treatments. They bring hope and often a reasonable quality of life to many children, but at present they cannot be regarded as curative procedures.

Part Two
Cardiac Problems in Infancy

Fetal diagnosis 5

Fetal cardiac diagnosis is by echocardiography. Fetal echocardiography developed in the 1980s and it is now possible to diagnose major congenital heart disease antenatally. This requires time and expertise, and detailed fetal echocardiography is concentrated in tertiary referral centres. Congenital heart disease can be detected using a four-chamber view of the heart at 18–20 weeks gestation. This view is not difficult to obtain and it is the practice in many obstetric centres to screen fetuses with a four-chamber view (Figure 5.1).

If there is an abnormality a referral will be made for definition of anatomy and cardiological counselling. This approach will detect hypoplastic left heart, hypoplastic right heart (i.e. pulmonary atresia without a VSD, tricuspid atresia and severe Ebstein's anomaly) and double-inlet ventricle (single ventricle, Figure 5.2), but it will miss outlet defects such as transposition of the great arteries, Fallot's tetralogy, double-outlet right ventricle and truncus arteriosus, which require more detailed scanning to detect reliably.

Minor congenital heart disease may not be detected, for example small VSDs and mild valve stenoses.

Atrial septal defects are of course part of the normal fetal circulation and postnatal atrial septal defect cannot be diagnosed from the prenatal scans. Similarly, a persistent ductus arteriosus cannot be predicted. Coarctation of the aorta can be very difficult to detect, although often there is right ventricular enlargement and the aorta-to-pulmonary-artery ratio is reduced. Sometimes valve stenosis can develop during pregnancy and for that reason a follow-up scan in high-risk pregnancies is usually performed at around 32 weeks. Occasionally, marked progression of heart disease is seen so that a hypoplastic left heart or right heart can develop from initial aortic or pulmonary valve stenosis.

Fetal heart failure results in pericardial and pleural effusions, ascites and generalized oedema (hydrops fetalis). Non-immune hydrops can be due to complete heart block, tachyarrhythmias and structural heart disease such as severe aortic stenosis and hypoplastic right heart.

The risk of fetal echocardiography is generally accepted to be minimal. Doppler examination increases the ultrasonic energy dose but is also considered to be safe. It is probably wise not to undertake extensive cardiac Doppler studies in early pregnancy and, when

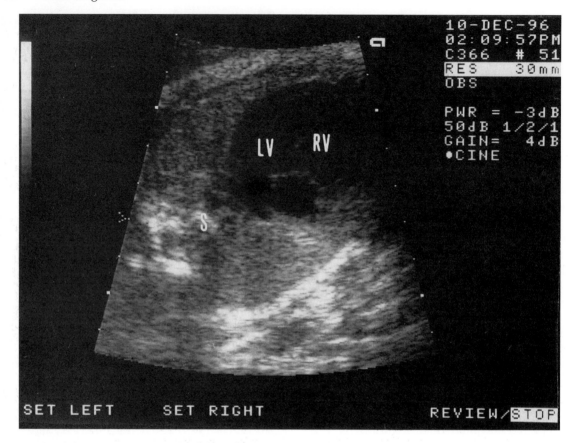

Figure 5.1 Fetal cardiac ultrasound scan. Normal four-chamber view. LV = left ventricle; RV = right ventricle; S = spine.

required, pulsed wave Doppler delivers more energy than colour Doppler and continuous wave delivers the lowest energy intensity of all.

Indications for cardiac scanning

Although abnormal screening scans are the most productive referral source of a new congenital heart disease there are other indications for fetal echocardiography (these are also discussed in Chapter 3).

- a family history of congenital heart disease in a first-degree relative;
- a family history of a single gene disorder with known cardiac involvement, e.g. Noonan's syndrome;
- exposure to teratogens in pregnancy;
- maternal diabetes (some centres would not consider this an indication for fetal echocardiography, but structural heart problems such as

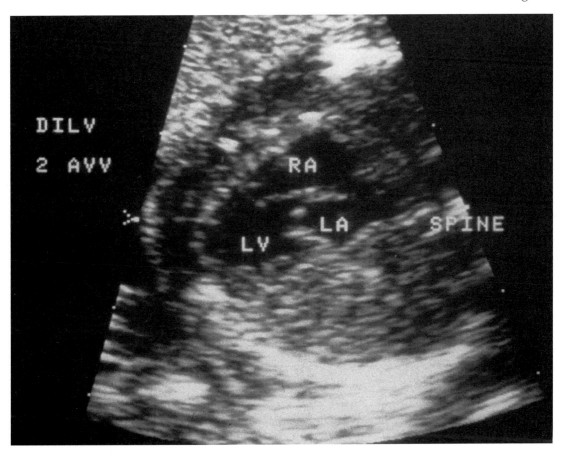

Figure 5.2   Fetal cardiac ultrasound scan. Four-chamber view showing both atria (LA and RA) opening into the left ventricle – double-inlet left ventricle. The right ventricle is extremely small and is not seen on this view. Reproduced by kind permission of Dr Ian Sullivan.

transposition, septal defects and coarctation are generally accepted to be more common and ventricular hypertrophy can also occur; see also Chapter 11);

- maternal systemic lupus erythematosus (SLE): this is associated with congenital complete heart block;
- other fetal anomaly: when one anomaly is seen on prenatal scanning it is usually wise to look for other abnormalities; for example, gastrointestinal abnormalities (such as diaphragmatic hernia and exomphalos) are well known to be associated with congenital heart disease but more subtle findings such as increased nuchal thickness are also indications of increased risk of cardiac disease;

- fetal chromosomal disorder: when an abnormality of the karyotype is detected a cardiac scan is often undertaken; for example, when trisomy 21 is found it can be helpful for counselling purposes to determine whether there is an associated atrioventricular septal defect;
- fetal arrhythmias.

Fetal arrhythmias   These can be brady- or tachyarrhythmias. The principal bradyarrhythmia is congenital complete heart block, which is diagnosed using M-mode echocardiography or Doppler. The rate of the atrial contraction can be determined and this is shown to be dissociated from ventricular contraction. The heart block is usually causally related to maternal anti-Ro antibody, which is often a marker of maternal SLE. Occasionally, congenital complete heart block is seen with structural heart disease such as congenitally corrected transposition. Most fetuses cope well with congenital complete heart block, but sometimes hydrops fetalis develops, although this is unusual if the rate is over 60/min. If the rate is less than 50/min assessments are made with a view to early delivery. If there is hydrops consideration should be given to delivery, which would be by caesarean section as monitoring for fetal distress is not possible. A transoesophageal pacing system is helpful to have nearby and the child should be delivered in a centre that can insert a permanent or temporary pacing system rapidly; chronotropic drugs such as isoprenaline may be helpful.

Referral for an irregular heart beat is common: most prove to be due to atrial ectopics, which can be diagnosed using M mode echocardiography or Doppler. These have a benign natural history and usually settle during pregnancy or in the early neonatal period. Rarely, they are associated with an atrial tachycardia. Ventricular ectopics are less common but also appear to be benign. Sometimes frequent paired atrial ectopics can be blocked and cause a slowing of the ventricular rate; again, this is a benign condition.

Supraventricular tachycardia is also seen. This is usually either from atrial flutter or from supraventricular tachycardia with a re-entrant circuit from an accessory pathway. If it is atrial flutter the atrial rate is very fast, over 400/min, but it is typically blocked 2 : 1 or more. Treatment is with maternal digoxin. Initially a loading dose is given and then maternal levels are monitored. Digoxin blocks the atrioventricular node and will slow the ventricular rate by preventing heart failure, but it probably does not induce sinus rhythm, the flutter reverting spontaneously. When there is a re-entrant tachycardia the rate is usually 220–300/min, with the atrial rate the same as the ventricular rate. Again, treatment is with maternal digoxin, which breaks the re-entrant circuit and restores sinus rhythm. If the fetus is hydropic flecainide is being increasingly used as it is a potent antiarrhythmic, but we remain concerned about its use when myocardial function is impaired. With resistant arrhythmias more unusual drugs are considered, but there is an increased risk of fetal loss.

Fetal ventricular tachycardia is uncommon but is sometimes seen when there is structural heart disease, particularly a ventricular tumour, the most common of which is a rhabdomyoma associated with tuberous sclerosis. Tumours are often multiple and grow rapidly in the last trimester, but if not causing a problem with inflow or outflow obstruction or an arrhythmia then there is no need for early delivery. They will often regress in infancy.

Management of prenatally diagnosed structural heart disease

Given the list of indications for fetal cardiac scanning it is clear that a rather different spectrum of abnormalities will be revealed to that seen postnatally (for example, there will be more fetuses with abnormal karyotype or other congenital anomaly). Conversely, if serious congenital heart disease is diagnosed at the 20-week scan it may be appropriate to offer amniocentesis for karyotyping. Cardiac counselling at this stage is crucial. In the UK termination of pregnancy for fetal anomalies is performed quite late in pregnancy, although often there is resistance to perform termination for congenital heart disease after 23 weeks. Therefore, when congenital heart disease is suspected definitive diagnosis and cardiac counselling are required rapidly. Given the current state of surgery for hypoplastic left ventricle in the UK, many parents will opt not to continue with the pregnancy after cardiac counselling. Similarly, many parents will not continue pregnancy when a child has an atrioventricular septal defect and trisomy 21. When parents do decide to continue with pregnancy they will need support during the remainder of pregnancy and ideally there should be delivery in a centre with access to obstetric/neonatal paediatrics and cardiac services, particularly for complex duct-dependent lesions, heart block and tachycardias. Fetal cardiac surgery has been pioneered in a few cardiac centres, and severe valve stenosis may be successfully treated with balloon dilatation, but at present prenatal cardiac surgery is not widely practised.

Fetal echocardiography is already having an impact on paediatrics and it is likely to continue to do so. Neonatal paediatricians are increasingly faced with prenatal diagnosis of serious congenital heart defects and the management plan will be made before the child is born. Furthermore, the spectrum of postnatal congenital heart disease may change, with some of the more severe abnormalities such as hypoplastic left or right heart becoming much less common.

The preterm neonate 6

Medical problems in the premature infant often have secondary cardio-vascular effects (Table 6.1).

PHYSIOLOGY

Patent ductus arteriosus

Only about 7% of combined ventricular output passes into the lungs in the fetus, with much of the right ventricular output crossing the arterial duct into the descending aorta. Patency of the arterial duct is maintained by circulating and locally produced prostaglandins *in utero*. The duct becomes less sensitive to prostaglandins and more sensitive to the constricting effect of oxygen as gestation progresses. At birth, increases in pulmonary arterial oxygen tension result in closure of the duct and consequently, as left atrial pressure rises, of the foramen ovale also. Preterm infants have a duct less sensitive to oxygen than at term and they may be subjected to hypoxaemia and acidosis as a result of respiratory disease. They may also have higher circulating levels of

Table 6.1 Cardiovascular sequelae of prematurity (all except PDA can be seen in term infants)

Condition	Comment
Patent ductus arteriosus	See text
Persistent pulmonary hypertension	With RDS, asphyxia, aspiration, congenital heart disease
Pneumopericardium	On positive pressure ventilation may cause tamponade
Thrombi and emboli	In association with long venous lines
Aortic thrombosis	From umbilical artery catheters
Infective endocarditis	Often not diagnosed in life; should be suspected with chronic signs of sepsis and multiple positive blood cultures
Right heart failure	In chronic lung disease

Table 6.2   Clinical features of delayed closure of ductus arteriosus

Context

- Not improving or deteriorating respiratory state, ventilator-dependent
- Apnoea
- Necrotizing enterocolitis
- Poor peripheral perfusion, metabolic acidosis

Specific signs

- Active precordium
- Bounding pulses: also caused by hypercapnia
- Murmur: continuous or systolic in pulmonary area, may be absent or intermittent

Investigations

- Chest X-ray: may show increasing cardiomegaly and pulmonary oedema; often unhelpful
- Electrocardiogram: rarely of value; only perform if another cardiac diagnosis suspected
- Echocardiography: very helpful in making diagnosis and assessing haemodynamic importance; essential before surgery, not essential before indomethacin if clinical picture very clear (features include direct imaging of the duct, Doppler assessment of the ductus, pulmonary artery and descending aorta flow patterns and volume overloading of the left heart, often indicated by left atrial:aortic ratio being increased above 1.3:1)

prostaglandins than term infants. All these influences act against the normal closure of the arterial duct, which may then contribute to the severity of respiratory and other problems.

CLINICAL PICTURE

Uncomplicated respiratory distress syndrome starts to improve after 48–72 hours. If this does not occur or starts and then deterioration occurs, delayed closure of the duct must be considered although other pulmonary pathology may also be the cause. Clinical features of delayed closure of the ductus in the premature are given in Table 6.2.

Antenatal steroid administration and cautious postnatal fluid regimes reduce the incidence of delayed closure of the ductus. Administration of indomethacin in the first 24–48 hours after birth reduces the incidence of symptomatic delayed closure of the ductus but detecting at that stage which babies are likely to develop symptomatic patent ductus arteriosus is not very reliable even if echocardiography including colour flow

Doppler is used (Plate 1). Early aggressive management is appropriate and, if there is any clinical doubt about the diagnosis, echocardiography is essential not only to confirm it but also to exclude the possibility of structural heart disease. The presence of a ductus without ventilator dependency or other major effects and not interfering with growth or weaning from oxygen need not be treated in the immediate weeks after birth. The natural history in the premature infant is of eventual spontaneous closure in many cases. The rationale for treatment is that there is evidence that, in the short term, dealing with symptomatic patent ductus reduces the need for respiratory support.

TREATMENT

An outline of treatment of symptomatic patent ductus is:

- optimize oxygen delivery (haemoglobin concentration and arterial oxygen tension);
- fluid restriction and diuretic, for a maximum of 24 hours only;
- Indomethacin if no contraindication, either:
  - 0.2 mg/kg IV 8–12–hourly × 3; or
  - 0.1 mg/kg IV daily × 6;
- Repeat indomethacin if:
  - short course used; and
  - some beneficial effect but only transient; and
  - no contraindication;
- surgery if indomethacin as outlined above fails or is contraindicated.

Indomethacin should be injected over 30 minutes to reduce its cerebral vasoconstriction effects, but near-infrared spectroscopy still shows very marked disturbance in cerebral haemodynamics even when the drug is given over 30 minutes. Fluid intake should be reduced by 20–25% around the time of drug administration. There is some evidence that administering dopamine or frusemide may counteract the fluid-retaining effect of indomethacin.

Symptomatic patent ductus arteriosus is found in 20–40% of infants of less than 1750 g birth weight. Indomethacin used as above will allow approximately 70% of these infants to avoid further therapy for symptomatic patent ductus and show at least short-term respiratory improvement. Long-term benefits in terms of time in oxygen, length of hospital stay and improved neurodevelopmental outcome have not clearly been demonstrated. The benefits of low-dose, longer-duration indomethacin are lower relapse rates and less disturbance in biochemical measures of renal function, but cerebral haemodynamics have not been examined with a 6-day course and the 3-day regime is the

Table 6.3   Indomethacin

Contraindications

- Renal failure (marked elevation or rapidly rising urea/creatinine concentrations)
- Bleeding or marked thrombocytopenia ($<50 \times 10^9$)
- Necrotizing enterocolitis or gastrointestinal haemorrhage

Side effects

- Transient oliguria and hyponatraemia
- Gastric haemorrhage, gastrointestinal perforation
- Transient hypertension if injected rapidly
- Reduces cerebral blood flow; significance unclear

more commonly used. Contraindications and side effects of the drug are listed in Table 6.3.

Other prostaglandin synthetase inhibitors have also been shown to be effective in closing the PDA, with some suggestion that ibuprofen does not disturb cerebral haemodynamics. However, experience with other drugs is less extensive and indomethacin remains the pharmacological treatment of choice. Surgical closure of the ductus should not be delayed if good improvement is not seen with medical management. Echocardiographic confirmation of the diagnosis is essential before surgery, which can be carried out with low morbidity and very low mortality in the neonatal unit at the surgical centre.

The pink neonate 7

Most cardiac conditions do not cause cyanosis and some conditions classified as cyanotic may cause only very mild or even unrecognized cyanosis in the newborn period. These are typically common mixing situations with unobstructed (and therefore high) pulmonary blood flow, such as unobstructed total anomalous pulmonary venous drainage, truncus arteriosus and univentricular atrioventricular connection (for example double-inlet left ventricle) without pulmonary stenosis. Also, if a non-cyanotic condition causes gross pulmonary oedema, cyanosis will be present but this will correct with oxygen therapy.

Introduction

All newborn babies are routinely examined and one sign looked for is a heart murmur. A murmur may be evidence of cardiac disease or it may be innocent. History and other features in cardiovascular examination are very important in the assessment of the cause of the murmur. ECG and chest X-ray may be useful but often will not help to distinguish innocent from pathological murmurs.

Murmurs

The commonest innocent murmur in the newborn period comes from the pulmonary artery bifurcation, as the branches are relatively hypoplastic at birth, having received only a small proportion of the cardiac output in fetal life. Characteristics of such murmurs are given in Table 7.1.

It is not certain but murmurs are probably not heard from the ductus arteriosus in normal newborn babies. A common and ultimately harmless murmur is that of tricuspid regurgitation, often associated with perinatal stress and minor T-wave changes in the left chest leads on ECG. Such murmurs are indistinguishable from those coming from small ventricular septal defects (VSDs) and indeed the lesions often coexist. Small VSDs often cause a murmur in the newborn period, but may not be associated with a murmur if the pulmonary resistance (and therefore the right ventricular pressure) is high, as there will be no pressure gradient between the ventricles. When the resistance falls, over the next few days, the murmur will become obvious. The apparent failure to detect a VSD murmur at an early neonatal check does cause concern to parents until the reason is explained.

Table 7.1   Innocent murnur in newborn infants

History	No symptoms
Examination	No other signs of cardiovascular disease

	Murmur	Mid-systolic
		Rarely louder than 2/6, never louder than 3/6
		Rough, high-pitched
		Maximum in pulmonary area
		Well heard upper back and both sides of chest
		Most gone by 3 months ⎫
		All disappeared by 6 months ⎬ in term infants ⎭

ECG, CXR normal

Echocardiogram (not essential for diagnosis) may show mild increase in blood velocity between main pulmonary artery and branches, may show patent foramen ovale

Table 7.2   Conditions associated with neonatal heart murmurs

- Obstructed lesions
  - Right or left ventricular outflow obstruction – valvar, sub- or supravalvar
  - Coarctation, particularly when duct closes
- Regurgitant lesions
  - Mitral regurgitation ⎫ may be a marker for heart muscle dysfunction
  - Tricuspid regurgitation ⎬ or part of a structural disorder
- Shunt lesions
  - ASD rarely causes murmur in the neonate
  - VSD, PDA may cause murmur, although not necessarily, particularly if large or if the pulmonary vascular resistance is high, as it is in the first few days of life; in the latter case the murmur may become apparent at a later check when the pulmonary resistance has fallen
  - In AVSD, AV valve regurgitation is more likely to cause the murmur than shunting as the defect is usually large with pressure equalization

Many serious heart abnormalities are associated with unimpressive or even no murmurs and large shunt lesions (such as a large VSD or an atrioventricular septal defect, where the ventricular pressures are equalized and flow across the hole is at low velocity) frequently are not accompanied by a murmur in the newborn period even if other, sometimes subtle, signs are present such as a dynamic precordium and abnormal heart sounds.

Groups of conditions which may present with or be characteristically associated with heart murmurs in the neonate are listed in Table 7.2.

The most important point about assessing an asymptomatic neonate with a murmur is to be sure that there is no duct-dependent structural heart disease, as such infants will collapse when the duct closes. In the absence of echocardiography the following are helpful in this assessment:

- definitely no symptoms;
- definitely pink (a hyperoxia test or pulse oximetry may help);
- strong synchronous femoral pulses felt over a period of 30 s;
- no hint of tachypnoea;
- normal postnatal weight loss (unexpected weight gain may represent early heart failure);
- normal heart sounds, no added sounds;
- murmur not best or only heard between scapulae (suggests coarctation); note distinction between this and pulmonary artery branch murmurs (Table 7.1);
- no difference between arm and leg blood pressures (occasionally this can be misleading, so too much emphasis should not be placed on normal values, particularly if the femoral pulses are abnormal);
- normal ECG and no cardiomegaly or pulmonary plethora on X-ray.

If doubt exists after working down this checklist a further period of observation in hospital is desirable if echocardiography is not available, although there should be a low threshold for referral to a cardiologist.

Heart failure

Poor feeding, breathlessness, grunting, clammy sweatiness and a worried appearance are reported in babies in heart failure. In the short term there will be excessive or unexplained weight gain in the context of poor feeding; failure to thrive is seen in the later neonatal period and beyond. Respiratory distress, tachycardia (unless heart block is present) and hepatomegaly are found on examination. Oedema is only rarely present but may be seen if the cause was active prior to delivery, when ascites and pleural effusions may also be found. A gallop rhythm may be heard and specific signs of the cardiac abnormality causing failure may be detected. Conditions presenting with neonatal heart failure are listed in Table 7.3.

Heart failure may also develop in some cyanotic conditions but in these circumstances it is not usually the presenting sign (see Table 8.4 in Chapter 8). Irrespective of cause there are management principles in neonatal heart failure.

- **Acute management:**
  - Ensure ventilation and oxygenation are adequate and avoid hyperoxia (which may increase left-to-right shunting).

Table 7.3   Conditions presenting with neonatal heart failure

Structural heart disease

- Left heart obstruction
  - Hypoplastic left heart syndrome
  - Interrupted aortic arch
  - Coarctation
  - Severe aortic stenosis

- Left to right shunt lesions
  - Rarely cause neonatal heart failure, except PDA in pre-term infants

Myocardial disease

- Myocarditis

- Cardiomyopathy
  - Hypertrophic – any cause
  - Dilated – any cause

Rhythm disturbance

- Supraventricular tachycardia
  - Atrioventricular re-entry
  - Atrial flutter

- Complete heart block
  - With structural heart disease
  - Without structural heart disease

Arteriovenous fistula (cerebral, hepatic)

Non-cardiac causes

- Anaemia

- Fluid overload

  - Consider prostaglandin if duct-dependent systemic circulation could be present (see below).
  - Diuretics (frusemide 1 mg/kg IV) give symptomatic relief.
  - Ensure blood glucose is maintained.
  - Treat anaemia, sepsis, electrolyte disturbance.
  - Consider cause.
  - Consider infusion of inotropes.
- **Chronic management** (when diagnosis or at least diagnostic group is known); see also p. 88.
  - Restrict fluids only if essential.
  - Optimize nutrition.
  - Frusemide oral/nasogastrically 1 mg/kg 8–12-hourly.
  - Maintain normal potassium by either spironolactone 1 mg/kg oral/nasogastrically 8–12-hourly or potassium chloride supplements.

- Angiotensin converting enzyme (ACE) inhibitors should be used with caution in neonates but are an effective treatment (see p. 88).
- Digoxin (maintenance 5 µg/kg oral/nasogastrically 12-hourly) is sometimes used but opinions vary on its merits and many are opposed to routine use.

Collapse

This may be overt shock, severe heart failure or severe hypoxaemia producing acidosis. Although collapse is considered in this chapter on the pink neonate it must be remembered that some cyanotic lesions can present with or progress to this condition and that duct-dependent systemic circulation (e.g. coarctation) can coexist with some cyanotic lesions (e.g. transposition with or without double-inlet left ventricle). Primary pathology outside the cardiovascular system can present with collapse; the following possibilities must be borne in mind.

- **Cardiac disease:**
  - Arrhythmia
  - Structural heart disease
  - Duct-dependent circulation, systemic or pulmonary
  - Heart muscle disease: primary (e.g. cardiac hypertrophy as in infant of diabetic mother or dilated cardiomyopathy); secondary (e.g. myocarditis, perinatal asphyxia)
- **Infection:** Septicaemia
- **Metabolic disease:** Inborn errors of metabolism
- **Neurological disease:** Birth asphyxia/trauma
- **Reduced circulating volume:**
  - Blood loss from any source
  - Dehydration for any reason
- **Respiratory disease:** Pneumothorax.

Structural heart disease usually produces collapse some days after birth as closure of the ductus arteriosus is the chief precipitating factor in many cases. History and examination are likely to rule out many of the causes listed above. Chest X-ray will often be helpful in reinforcing the decision that a cardiac cause is or is not present; cardiac disease causing collapse is likely to produce cardiomegaly or pulmonary oligaemia on X-ray, or, in the case of obstructed TAPVD, a normal heart size with fine opacification of lung fields that can be hard to distinguish from RDS.

In all causes the emergency management has much in common by way of general resuscitation, i.e. dealing with:

- ventilatory failure
- hypoglycaemia

Table 7.4 Lesions likely to present or deteriorate markedly when the ductus arteriosus closes (ASD = atrial septal defect; VSD = ventricular septal defect)

- Duct-dependent systemic circulation
  - Coarctation
  - Hypoplastic left heart syndrome
  - Aortic valve atresia
  - Interrupted aortic arch
- Duct-dependent pulmonary circulation ⎫
  - Pulmonary atresia
    with intact ventricular septum
    with VSD (but no aortopulmonary
    communicating arteries)   cyanotic lesions, see
  - Critical pulmonary stenosis   Chapter 18
  - Tricuspid atresia (unless large VSD)
- Transposition without large ASD or VSD ⎭

- hypoxaemia
- acidosis
- reduced circulating volume
- infection.

There are a number of specific points to note if cardiac disease is suspected.

- **Structural duct-dependent congenital heart disease.** If one of these lesions is suspected (Table 7.4), prostaglandin should be commenced and if the diagnosis is correct an improvement in peripheral pulses (duct-dependent systemic circulation) or in oxygenation (duct-dependent pulmonary circulation) is likely within 30–60 minutes.

  If this happens, many of the other theoretical possibilities do not need to be pursued and assisted ventilation for hypoxaemia may be seen not to be needed. For further information on prostaglandin see p. 83 and for details of specific conditions see Chapter 16 (duct-dependent systemic circulation) and Chapter 18 (duct-dependent pulmonary circulation).
- If a **dysrhythmia** is the cause of the collapse, treatment of the rhythm disturbance will restore blood pressure and vital organ and peripheral perfusion. Infusions of plasma expanders may be harmful as well as ineffective in dysrhythmias.

Dysrhythmias   Abnormalities of rhythm may be detected coincidentally in newborn infants with other illnesses, in asymptomatic babies at routine assessments or because of illness directly attributable to the rhythm. Unlike adult dysrhythmias, symptoms are usually of heart failure, even with simple supraventricular tachycardias, probably because of a rate-dependent cardiac output in the neonatal period. Occasionally, sudden episodes of collapse or apparent fits may be manifestations of neonatal arrhythmias. Management depends on what the rhythm is and what if any haemodynamic disturbance is occurring or could develop. For further consideration of rhythm disturbances see Chapter 14.

Pulse abnormalities

Many structural heart lesions may be associated with abnormalities in pulse volume or character but in the newborn period the lesion commonly presenting with an abnormal pulse is coarctation of the aorta, when absent or weak femoral pulses in an asymptomatic infant are often the first clue to the diagnosis. Reduced femoral pulses are an indication for cardiological referral and although careful blood pressure measurements in arms and legs can give information about a pressure gradient, it can be misleading. Similarly, ECG and chest X-ray may offer further proof of underlying cardiac disease but a normal ECG and chest X-ay do not rule out coarctation and even with echocardiography coarctation can be difficult to rule out before the ductus arteriosus starts to close.

The blue neonate 8

The clinical problem of a blue newborn baby is common: in most cases there is an airway or respiratory problem. Cyanotic episodes in newborn infants are less likely to be due to cardiac disease than is sustained cyanosis. Central cyanosis can be readily differentiated from acrocyanosis and facial petechiae (traumatic cyanosis), both of which are common and rarely of significance. A polycythaemic infant may look centrally cyanosed but have normal arterial oxygen tension; this can usually be confirmed by pulse oximetry or transcutaneous oxygen tension monitoring without needing to resort to arterial blood sampling. Table 8.1 gives the features of different groups of causes of central cyanosis in the newborn.

Introduction

Table 8.1 Causes of neonatal central cyanosis

Cause	*Comment*
Respiratory disease	More likely in preterm infants, who are likely to have respiratory distress Often improved by increasing oxygen concentration
Cardiac disease	Most are term infants May be otherwise well May have other cardiovascular signs Unlikely to be improved by oxygen
Persistent pulmonary hypertension	May have been asphyxiated Associated with respiratory and less commonly cardiac disease Cyanosis variable
Methaemoglobinaemia	Very rare; may have family history or maternal exposure to oxidizing agents Well
Cerebral disease Hypoglycaemia Hypocalcaemia	Mediated *via* respiratory or pulmonary vascular derangement

Table 8.2   Tests to distinguish causes of cyanosis

	Cardiac	*Respiratory*
Chest X-ray	May be normal May have abnormal heart size or shape Vascular markings may be abnormal Lung changes can be non-specific (obstructed TAPVD may resemble hyaline membrane	Rarely normal Often diagnostic
ECG	May be normal Occasionally helpful	Usually normal
Arterial blood gas	Oxygen low Carbon dioxide normal/low	Oxygen low Carbon dioxide normal/high
Hyperoxia test	Usually fail	Often pass (at least in early stages)

Evaluation   Often history and examination allows differentiation between the causes of cyanosis, in practice the need to distinguish between cardiac and respiratory causes is the commonly encountered situation. If doubt exists after history and examination a number of simple tests usually suffice, as shown in Table 8.2.

The hyperoxia or nitrogen washout test is simply a structured way of evaluating the response to oxygen, and examination of the blood gas chart of an ill baby may provide the same information without formally conducting the test. It should not be performed on infants for whom even short periods of hyperoxia may be a risk factor for retinopathy. The hyperoxia test was originally described to help distinguish cardiac and respiratory causes of cyanosis if cardiac catheterization would otherwise have been needed. The baby was placed in an inspired oxygen concentration of 85% or more for over 10 minutes and if the right radial artery oxygen tension had risen above 20 kPa the baby was likely to have respiratory disease, although some common mixing cardiac conditions will also achieve this, e.g. total anomalous pulmonary venous drainage and double inlet ventricle. Failure of the hyperoxia test makes cyanotic congenital heart disease more likely, although infants with severe respiratory disease and those with persistent pulmonary hypertension will also fail. In infants for whom this test is necessary to make the distinction, there will be other reasons for knowing the arterial blood gas values, although transcutaneous oxygen tension monitoring can be used providing the electrode is on the right upper chest (i.e. preductal) and it does not lift off the skin in the headbox thereby giving a spectacular but false pass.

Two additional uses of the hyperoxia test principle which can be done with a transcutaneous monitor are:

- if it is unclear whether a dusky baby is truly desaturated; normal and mildly abnormal oxygen tension in air may be hard to distinguish but the response to breathing an increased oxygen concentration will usually clarify this;
- a failed hyperoxia test may warn that a well baby with an apparently straightforward cardiac abnormality has in fact a more complex one.

Pulse oximeters are widely used in neonatal nurseries. A baby cannot pass the hyperoxia test with a pulse oximeter as a saturation of 100% may be associated with an arterial oxygen tension of 7–8 kPa or 45 kPa because of the shape of the haemoglobin-oxygen dissociation curve. However, failure of a hyperoxia test using an oximeter (i.e. failure to increase saturation to 90% or more) is significant and may be of value in the two additional uses for the test given above.

Most cases of cyanotic congenital heart disease that require early intervention for cyanosis have a resting saturation of less than 80% and do not increase saturations to above 90% in 100% oxygen. Some cases of common mixing can have higher saturations. There is the theoretical risk of promoting closure of the ductus arteriosus during a hyperoxia test and for this reason infants should be observed during it.

Cyanotic congenital heart disease

The three groups of structural congenital heart disease causing cyanosis are listed in Table 8.3.

Some cardiac conditions can be placed in more than one category. Heart failure rarely causes cyanosis unless pulmonary oedema is gross but some cyanotic conditions are associated with heart failure. These are listed in Table 8.4. These neonates have a raised respiratory rate and therefore this sign cannot be used to confirm respiratory rather than cardiac disease, although a well infant with severe cyanosis and a normal respiratory rate is likely to have cardiac disease.

The immediate management of cyanotic congenital heart disease does not depend on a specific diagnosis being made, although this can sometimes be done with accuracy without echocardiography. The important immediate concerns are as follows.

- Optimize general condition of infant.
- Ensure respiration is adequate.
- Decide whether prostaglandin is required.

Table 8.3   Classification of cyanotic congenital heart disease

Category	Examples	Comments
Right to left shunts	Tricuspid atresia Pulmonary atresia with intact ventricular septum Critical pulmonary stenosis	Cyanosis recognized in early newborn gets worse as duct shuts
	Tetralogy of Fallot	Minority of cases blue in newborn period
Common mixing	Total anomalous pulmonary venous drainage	Often only midly cyanosed, more so if pulmonary veins obstructed
	Double inlet ventricle	Degree of cyanosis depends on degree of pulmonary stenosis
	Truncus arteriosus	
Transposition		Degree of cyanosis depends on number/size of shunt lesions and on presence or not of pulmonary stenosis

Table 8.4   Lesions in which cyanosis and heart failure often coexist

- TGA
  - with large VSD and PDA
  - with coarctation

- Truncus arteriosus

- Double inlet ventricle

- Tricuspid atresia
  - with coarctation and TGA
  - with large VSD

- Hypoplastic left heart

- Total anomalous pulmonary venous drainage

In general the greater the lung blood flow the worse the failure and the less blue the infant
Pulmonary stenosis in addition to one of these lesions produces more severe cyanosis but less or no failure

- Assess infant for underlying syndrome or congenital abnormalities in other systems.
- Give antibiotic after blood culture if the possibility of serious infection exists.

- Sort out details of transfer to cardiac centre.
- Take time to communicate with parents.

Prostaglandin E series will reopen or keep open the ductus arteriosus, which will increase lung blood flow, and should be given to:

- very blue infants (P_AO_2 3.5 kPa or less, saturations 70%), who will become acidotic;
- those who are getting bluer (usually associated with ductal closure);
- those who have metabolic acidosis;
- those who are shocked;

and should be seriously considered in those with oligaemic lung fields on X-ray.

Prostaglandin will usually improve oxygenation or prevent deterioration in those with obstruction to blood flow through the right heart and in transposition. Left atrial pressure rises if lung blood flow is increased and in transposition this will cause increased shunting of oxygenated blood into the right atrium (and hence right ventricle and aorta), providing an adequate foramen ovale or atrial septal defect exists. Prostaglandin E_1 can be used intravenously; E_2 is absorbed from the gastrointestinal tract as well as being available for intravenous use. It makes sense to have only one preparation available and E_2 is the appropriate one.

There has been much discussion about dosage of the two preparations in the past. The regime given below is for prostaglandin E_2 but similar intravenous doses can be used for prostaglandin E_1.

Prostaglandin E_2 intravenously 0.005 µg/kg/min (5 ng/kg/min) may be increased stepwise to 0.05 µg/kg/min if no effect is seen and no side effects are encountered. Such an increase is rarely necessary; it is often possible to reduce the maintenance dose from the starting dose (avoid flushing the drip as this may cause apnoea). The oral/nasogastric dose is 25 µg/kg/h hourly initially. The dose may need to be doubled. For long-term use it can be made 2- or even 4-hourly.

Side effects of prostaglandin include apnoea, jitteriness, convulsions, pyrexia, diarrhoea, fever and flushing and are improved by stopping the infusion and restarting at a lower dose. Serious side effects from gastric administration are very uncommon. The possibility of apnoea should be considered prior to commencing an infusion, particularly if transfer is considered, and a prostaglandin intravenous line should never be flushed as this can precipitate apnoea.

Persistent pulmonary hypertension of the newborn

This condition (also called persistent fetal circulation) may be associated with a variety of causes, such as birth asphyxia with or without meconium pneumonitis, or any type of respiratory disease or pulmonary hypoplasia such as occurs with diaphragmatic hernia. Echocardiography is sometimes required to exclude cyanotic congenital heart disease. Also, the right-to-left shunting associated with pulmonary hypertension can be of greater volume when there is a large septal defect e.g. an atrioventricular septal defect, as in Down's syndrome, and such children can be profoundly cyanosed. Helpful clinical features pointing to the diagnosis of persistent fetal circulation include:

- history of fetal distress, including meconium staining;
- need for active resuscitation after birth, including the presence of meconium below the vocal cords;
- concurrent respiratory and neurological signs;
- radiological evidence of aspiration pneumonitis or other severe pulmonary pathology;
- transient improvements in oxygenation, particularly with respiratory alkalosis obtained by assisted ventilation;
- saturations in the right hand 4% or more above a simultaneous reading from the foot (suggesting right-to-left ductal shunting). This is also seen with some cardiac lesions, such as interrupted aortic arch or severe coarctation.

Management consists of:

- normalizing blood sugar, calcium and magnesium;
- correcting polycythaemia;
- hyperventilating to respiratory alkalosis (pH approximately 7.5) in high inspired oxygen;
- supporting blood pressure with colloid and inotropes;
- specific pulmonary vasodilators, i.e. oxygen and inhaled nitric oxide; endotracheal tolazoline has been tried and is possibly effective;
- non-specific vasodilating drugs such as tolazoline 0.5 mg/kg as a bolus followed by 0.5–1 mg/kg/h or prostacyclin 2–20 ng/kg/min. These will cause systemic hypotension and so continuous invasive blood pressure monitoring is essential to enable treatment with colloid and inotrope to be given. Both drugs have been implicated in a bleeding tendency.

Specific cyanotic heart lesions

See Chapter 18.

The older infant 9

Introduction

The patterns of congenital and acquired heart disease in infancy but after the newborn period are not substantially different from those discussed in earlier chapters with respect to the neonate. There are, however, a number of variations worth pointing out and these will be considered under the same headings as those used when referring to newborn infants.

THE BLUE INFANT

Distinguishing cardiac from non-cardiac cyanosis in infancy is based on the same criteria as with the newborn. Respiratory disease causing cyanosis is usually very acute in onset and easily recognized, with severe respiratory distress. Occasionally, confusion arises when an infant with previously unrecognized desaturation develops an intercurrent respiratory illness, for example bronchiolitis. Physical examination, ECG and CXR usually alert to the presence of cardiac disease. Cyanotic congenital heart disease presenting after the newborn period will have escaped earlier recognition because lung blood flow was high (e.g. complex pulmonary atresia with large collateral arteries), making cyanosis mild, or because obstruction to lung blood flow was progressive (e.g. Fallot's tetralogy). Conditions presenting or coming to be recognized as cyanotic after the newborn period are listed in Table 9.1. Lesions in the last two groups in the table commonly develop into heart failure.

Many cyanotic conditions presenting in the newborn period will remain cyanosed in infancy having had palliative interventions although some will have been corrected such as transposition and total anomalous pulmonary venous drainage. Certain points of management are common to all cyanotic infants (Table 9.2).

Hypercyanotic spells often occur on waking from sleep. They are rare in the newborn period but if they are going to develop are usually present by the end of infancy. The infant starts to cry and looks bluer than usual. When crying stops, however, colour does not return to normal and the infant appears drowsy or even unresponsive, with deep acidotic respiration. The pathophysiological process involved in spells is

Table 9.1   Cyanotic conditions in the older infant

Group	Example	Comment
Right to left shunt	Tetralogy of Fallot	1. Commonly subvalvar right ventricular outflow obstruction is mild at birth and progresses, resulting in cyanosis. 2. Less common with pulmonary atresia and major aortopulmonary arteries, resulting in high pulmonary blood flow and therefore mild cyanosis; these infants have continuous murmurs over both sides of the chest
	Pulmonary arteriovenous malformations	Very rare, usually not recognized until later childhood
Common mixing	Truncus arteriosus	Cyanosis is often mild and may not be obvious
	Double inlet left ventricle	Degree of pulmonary stenosis determines level of cyanosis
	Unobstructed TAPVD	
Transposition	Transposition with large VSD	Without pulmonary obstruction, VSD allows good mixing of blood

still contested but probably involves a sudden increase in subvalvar right ventricular outflow obstruction, which is attributed to cardiac muscle spasm (infundibular spasm). The immediate first aid treatment out of hospital involves intermittent knee chest positioning (for up to 2 min at a time) to increase systemic vascular resistance and help to reduce the right-to-left shunt. In hospital intravenous propranolol is given which reduces infundibular spasm (0.05 mg/kg intravenously) or intravenous phenylephrine (0.01–0.02 mg/kg intravenously), which increases peripheral vascular resistance and systemic blood pressure, thereby reducing intracardiac shunting. Intravenous morphine is sometimes given for analgesia and sedation. If these measures have not worked, much heavier sedation or general anaesthesia with assisted ventilation are very occasionally required. A spell should always be discussed with a cardiologist as it may be an indication for prompt cardiac surgery.

Table 9.2 Management of cyanotic infants

Topic	Comment	Action
Avoid iron deficiency	Microcytosis decreases red cell deformability and thus increases blood viscosity	Avoid late weanng and thereby ensure adequate iron intake Check haematocrit and blood film at 6 months
Avoid dehydration	Likely to be polycythaemic even when well hydrated	Seek help early in intercurrent illnesses
Ensure good weight gain	At risk of failure to thrive	Close community follow-up
Endocarditis risk	Ensure family and health professionals aware	
Influenza risk		Immunize
Other infection risk	Most cases DiGeorge syndrome Asplenia (in right isomerism)	Standard immunization see p. 38 see p. 46
Recurrence risk	Will be increased	Counsel family
Identify if at risk of hypercyanotic spells	Conditions with muscular pulmonary outflow obstruction, e.g. tetralogy of Fallot	Discuss with parents and family doctor

Heart failure

Typically, shunt lesions do not cause failure until 2–3 months of age. Secundum ASDs very rarely cause heart failure; primum type ASDs (partial AVSD) may cause heart failure in infancy, particularly if atrioventricular valve regurgitation is marked. Complete AVSD, large VSDs and PDAs may all cause heart failure; if they do not it is for one of three reasons.

- Pulmonary vascular resistance falls insufficiently to allow great increase in lung blood flow; this may result in the severity of the lesion being unrecognized and progressive irreversible pulmonary vascular changes progressing unnoticed to Eisenmenger haemodynamics (p. 134).
- Lesions are small; this is virtually never the case in complete AVSD and must never be assumed.
- Pulmonary outflow obstruction is present (in VSD and AVSD).

Other causes of heart failure after the newborn period include arrhythmias, heart muscle disease (congenital or acquired) and chronic lung disease (cor pulmonale).

Acute treatment of heart failure is as described on pp. 73–4. Chronic treatment of heart failure includes the following.

- **Diuretic**: frusemide (1 mg/kg 8–12-hourly, may increase to 2 mg/kg/ dose) and either spironolactone (1 mg/kg 8–12-hourly up to 2 mg/kg/ dose) or potassium supplement (start at 1 mmol/kg 8–12-hourly). Keep plasma K$^+$ at 3.5–4.5 mmol/l.
- **Digoxin** is still used by some cardiologists. Give 4–5 µg/kg 12-hourly and adjust according to blood levels 6 hours post-dose after 5–7 days treatment, unless a loading regime is used, which is not indicated in the treatment of heart failure.
- **ACE inhibitor** – captopril: start at 0.1 mg/kg 8-hourly and build up in several steps to 1.5–2 mg/kg/d in three doses. Measure blood pressure every 15 minutes after the first dose and after each increased dose until the fall has reached trough and started to rise. Reduce dose if symptomatic hypotension or systolic pressure falls by more than 25%. Watch for hyperkalaemia (reduce potassium or give potassium-sparing diuretics) and elevation of creatinine (reduce ACE inhibitor dose). Adverse effects will be worse if the infant is already dehydrated by diuretics. Liver function derangement and neutropenia can occur.
- Avoid sodium supplements if possible by controlling hyponatraemia with altered diuretic dose.
- Adequate calorie intake is essential, so avoid fluid restriction if possible: put additives in feeds. Nasogastric feeding may be necessary. Overnight infusions and gastrostomy insertion should be employed according to local experience, although gastrostomy has drawbacks; i.e. nearness of wound to sternotomy site and possibility of skin sepsis or colonization as a risk for cardiac surgical wound infection or endocarditis source.

Heart failure preventing adequate weight gain is an important factor that influences the timing of surgical intervention in structural heart disease.

Heart murmur   Asymptomatic heart murmurs in infancy can be a presentation of any obstructive, shunt or regurgitant lesion, or may be innocent. Innocent murmurs are subject to the same considerations as in the newborn when the infant is under 6 months, and as in the older child when the infant is older than 6 months. See Chapter 10 for further discussion.

Part Three
Cardiac Problems in the Older Child

Cardiology in the paediatric outpatient department 10

One of the most common referrals in paediatric clinics is that of a child with a heart murmur that has been noticed by a primary care physician. The prevalence of innocent murmurs is varied in published studies (6–90%), but it is generally accepted that they are very common and a reasonable estimate would be that one in ten children has an innocent murmur at a pre-school medical.

When faced with a new referral it is important to take a full history and complete cardiac examination as detailed in the earlier section. Having excluded serious cardiac pathology it is sensible to consider whether the murmur is innocent. In fact, there are several different types of innocent murmur so it is helpful to consider whether the murmur fits into one of these groups.

STILL'S MURMUR

Still described this murmur in the early part of the 20th century. It is frequently heard in children between the ages of 4 and 6 and therefore will often be detected when a school entry check is being undertaken. The cause of the murmur is unknown, but it is probably of left ventricular origin, and is produced as blood is ejected through the rather cylindrically shaped left ventricle of young children and is easily heard in this age group because there is less dense tissue between the heart and the stethoscope than in adults. It accounts for most of the murmur referrals to paediatricians. It is usually best heard between the left sternal edge and the apex and there is limited radiation. It is low-pitched and has a rather musical or vibratory quality. Although it is short, there is a crescendo–decrescendo character in mid systole. It is usually grade 1 or 2/6. Typically there is postural variation and the murmur is softer when the child stands up. Like all innocent murmurs it is louder when the cardiac output is increased. Still's murmur often disappears by puberty, although it can persist into adult life.

THE VENOUS HUM

The venous hum is, like Still's murmur, extremely common. In fact, fewer are referred to paediatricians as many primary care physicians recognize the venous hum. Although it is usually most prevalent in a pre-school age, it is sometimes heard in older children. Unlike all other innocent murmurs it has a diastolic component, being a continuous systolic/diastolic murmur. It is usually best heard below the clavicles, although sometimes it can be heard over a slightly wider area. The murmur is abolished by compression of the jugular vein or by lying the child down with the neck flexed and, as expected, it is loudest when the child is doing the opposite, i.e. standing with the neck extended.

PULMONARY FLOW MURMUR

This murmur is typically loudest in the pulmonary area and does not have the musical quality of a Still's murmur: the pitch is slightly higher, although it is still crescendo–decrescendo. There is postural variation, as in Still's murmur. Pulmonary flow murmurs are uncommon in young children, although they are quite common in adolescents and young adults. They are more common in individuals with straight posture ('straight back syndrome') and may only be heard when the cardiac output is high, e.g. after exercise, with a fever or during pregnancy. It can be hard to distinguish a pulmonary flow murmur from a small atrial septal defect or mild pulmonary stenosis, so it is important to listen for normal splitting of the second heart sound and to ensure that there is no ejection click.

NECK BRUITS

Like pulmonary flow murmurs, these are uncommon in young children, being more frequent in adolescence. It is sometimes hard to distinguish these bruits from mild aortic stenosis, but usually a neck bruit is not well heard in the aortic area, is maximal above the clavicle and there is no click or suprasternal thrill. A further useful trick is that shoulder hyperextension or subclavian artery compression will often abolish the murmur.

PULMONARY MURMUR OF THE NEWBORN

This murmur is probably caused by the change in flow patterns after birth when the relatively small fetal pulmonary arteries suddenly have to cope with all the cardiac output. It is typically short and harsh and audible at the sternal borders. Unlike the other innocent murmurs it can be heard over the back. It almost invariably disappears by 6 months of age. Important stenoses of the branch pulmonary arteries are typically longer systolic murmurs with wider radiation over both lung fields at the back and are typically associated with maternal rubella, Alagille's and Williams syndromes.

FURTHER INVESTIGATION OF MURMURS

Many paediatricians feel that a good history and physical examination are all that is required to diagnose innocent murmurs. If the diagnosis is positive, no further investigations are ordered, no follow-up is arranged and infectious endocarditis prevention measures are not recommended. Unfortunately, there are certain abnormalities that can be hard to distinguish from innocent murmurs. For example, hypertrophic cardio-myopathy and small VSDs can resemble Still's murmurs, while mild pulmonary stenosis and small ASDs cause quiet murmurs in the pulmo-nary area. Therefore it is common practice to order chest X-rays and ECGs, although often they do not help in distinguishing normal from abnormal murmurs. Many paediatricians adopt a conservative ap-proach with an annual review for any slightly atypical innocent mur-murs. When there is any doubt it is wise to obtain a cardiological opinion with a view to good-quality echocardiography, this has the advantage of abolishing the need for annual review and antibiotic prophylaxis if all is normal. It may occasionally reveal an unexpected significant lesion.

Follow up of congenital heart disease in clinic

Paediatricians usually follow up a large number of children with congenital heart disease in clinic.

There are a number of areas of management that are common and help to provide a structure to follow-up. It is very important that the children and parents are all educated about general matters (Figure 10.1) and in particular about endocarditis preventative measures (Fig-ure 10.2).

They should be made aware of the need for antibiotic cover for dental or surgical procedures and skin sepsis, e.g. infected chickenpox vesicles. Ear-piercing should be discouraged, as the holes often become infected. Booklets on the importance of dental care are available and antibiotic prophylaxis cards are supplied by the British Heart Founda-tion (Figure 10.2). The outpatient clinic also provides important oppor-tunities to prepare children for planned admissions (Figure 10.3)

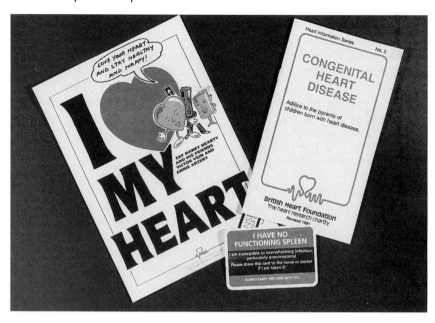

Figure 10.1   Educational literature. Examples of general educational literature for patients and families from the British Heart Foundation. We are grateful for their permission to reproduce.

For children with cyanosis it is worthwhile recording oxygen saturations with a pulse oximeter. Haemoglobin and PCV should also be monitored and venesection undertaken if necessary (as discussed in the adolescent section).

The ECG is a very useful investigation. When there is significant valve stenosis it will show evidence of increasing hypertrophy or even ventricular strain and with a large VSD the left ventricular voltages will increase progressively as the shunt increases. Apart from voltage or repolarization changes, it is useful to check the ECG regularly in postoperative patients to ensure that they remain in sinus rhythm and that there is no evidence of heart block. In more complex patients it is quite common to perform occasional 24 hour ambulatory ECGs, e.g. in tetralogy of Fallot or total cavopulmonary connection and also in patients with cardiomyopathy. It is rather controversial as to whether any tachyarrhythmia found on 24 hour monitoring should be treated, and there is even some controversy about whether asymptomatic bradyarrhythmias should be treated. The general feeling is that there is prognostic value in defining abnormalities on ambulatory tapes and that a decision on treatment should be discussed with the child's cardiologist.

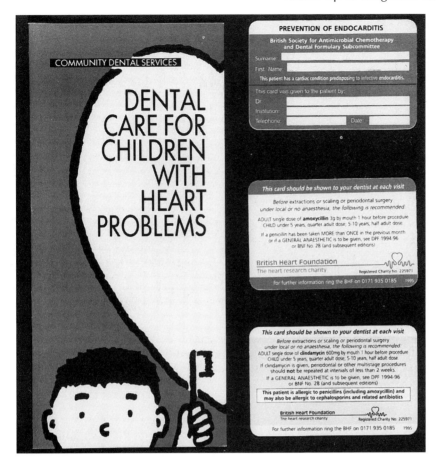

Figure 10.2   Educational literature. Literature on infective endocarditis. Reproduced with permission of Oxford Community Dental Services and the British Heart Foundation.

Chest X-rays are often used in follow-up of congenital heart disease although they are rarely necessary at every clinic attendance and have been rather superseded by echocardiography. This is extremely helpful in outpatient follow-up and increasingly paediatricians have access to the equipment.

Anticoagulation is usually managed in specific clinics, although the parameters should be defined by the child's cardiologist. For example, the INR is often maintained at a higher level in children with prosthetic valves than in those who are anticoagulated after a total cavopulmonary connection. Aspirin is commonly used as an intermediate anticoagulant, e.g. after Blalock shunts and sometimes after a cavopulmonary connection.

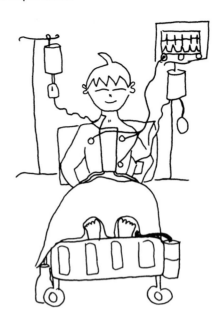

Figure 10.3   Educational literature. Picture for colouring to help prepare children for future cardiac surgery. Reproduced by kind permission of Neila Chrisp and Oxford Medical Illustration.

The need for exercise limitation is appropriately discussed in the outpatient setting. The majority of children with congenital heart disease (e.g. VSDs, ASDs and mild valve disease) can exercise freely, but there are a few subgroups in whom strenuous exertion should be avoided. These are those with:

- significant ventricular outflow obstruction, particularly aortic stenosis;
- cardiomyopathy, probably of any type;
- some arrhythmias, e.g. ventricular tachycardia, or any that have caused severe symptoms;
- Eisemenger's syndrome/pulmonary hypertension;
- Marfan's syndrome with a dilated aortic root;
- systemic hypertension.

All these children should be encouraged to play and even to take part in gentle sport, but competitive sport, isometric exercise (e.g. weight lifting) and extreme exertion should be avoided. Swimming should be accompanied in these high-risk groups. Children with complex congenital heart disease can often take part in some sport and their level of fitness may improve significantly; schools may need covering letters explaining realistic aims. Aggressive contact sports, risking a blow to the chest, should be avoided if there is an anterior homograft (e.g. after a Rastelli operation), or a pacemaker, with anticoagulation and for a few months after cardiac surgery.

Cardiomyopathy 11

As the name suggests, cardiomyopathy indicates disease of the myocardium. This can be primary/idiopathic, or secondary, where the cause is known. Characterization of the primary cardiomyopathies at metabolic, genetic and molecular levels has resulted in a blurring of the borders between primary and secondary cardiomyopathies. An important part of the management of childhood cardiomyopathies involves a search for a primary cause and this tends to be more extensive than that undertaken in adult patients with cardiomyopathy.

The primary cardiomyopathies can be further subgrouped into three types according to structure and function: dilated, hypertrophic and restrictive.

Dilated cardiomyopathy

This is characterized by an echocardiographic appearance of dilatation of the left or both ventricular cavities with reduced contractility. It is the commonest of the cardiomyopathies in childhood and is the main reason for children to present to paediatricians with newly diagnosed cardiac failure after infancy. It is also the most common indication for cardiac transplantation in paediatric practice.

PHYSICAL SIGNS

There is often evidence of heart failure, with tachycardia, tachypnoea and elevated jugular venous pressure. A gallop rhythm is common and a murmur of mitral regurgitation may be audible.

INVESTIGATION

Chest X-ray

The chest X-ray will demonstrate cardiomegaly, and often pulmonary oedema.

ECG

The ECG may demonstrate some broadening of the QRS complex and there may be evidence of ventricular strain, with T wave changes. The left ventricular voltages are usually increased. If they are markedly increased the diagnosis of endocardial fibroelastosis is considered, although this may not be a distinct entity but part of the spectrum of dilated cardiomyopathy. Ischaemic changes suggest an anomalous origin of the left coronary artery from the pulmonary artery.

24-hour ECG

This is helpful to exclude an incessant tachycardia, which may have been the primary cause of the cardiomyopathy. The heart rate will be inappropriately fast with little variation and often the P waves have an unusual axis and morphology. It is also important to document secondary arrhythmias in dilated cardiomyopathy, such as ventricular tachycardia and atrial flutter. Even if they are asymptomatic the documentation may help in defining the prognosis.

Echocardiography

This remains the most important investigation. Left ventricular function is usually assessed from fractional shortening (the product of left ventricular internal dimension in diastole minus left ventricular internal dimension in systole divided by left ventricular internal dimension in diastole, expressed as a percentage). Ejection fraction (which is a volumetric calculation) is also used, although it is arguably less accurate. The left ventricular internal dimension in diastole is increased and there are standard charts for normal values. Dilated cardiomyopathy can be familial in some cases, principally dominantly inherited with heterogeneous gene loci in the few families in whom it has been mapped. Routine screening of families is controversial and needs to handled sensitively. It is probably not indicated during the initial phase of investigations.

Endocardial fibroelastosis is characterized by focal thickening of the endocardium of the left ventricle, and also the left atrium and left-side valves. This appearance is also seen secondary to obstruction of the left ventricular outflow tract or aorta. The echocardiogram demonstrates very bright endocardial echo. Our opinion is that this appearance in dilated cardiomyopathy is secondary to the disease process rather than representing a specific disease entity, but opinions vary. It has been postulated that endocardial fibroelastosis is caused by the mumps virus and that the decreasing incidence in America is related to the use of MMR vaccine.

MYOCARDITIS

Paediatricians are often concerned that a new case of dilated cardio-myopathy could be myocarditis, as both present with heart failure and echocardiographic images are similar. Firstly, this is a problem because immunosuppression treatment has been advocated for myocarditis, although recent evidence suggests there is little role for this. The second area of concern is that myocarditis may improve spontaneously when the precipitating cause is removed and therefore a decision to refer a new patient for cardiac transplantation should be deferred until myo-carditis has been excluded. Unfortunately, it is very difficult to diagnose myocarditis. Recent viral infection is very common in paediatric prac-tice and a rising viral titre on paired serology will not enable an early diagnosis to be made. Viruses often implicated in myocarditis are Coxsackie, ECHO, influenza, parainfluenza, HIV (which can lead to a chronic dilated cardiomyopathy), mumps, rubella and measles, al-though other viral and non-viral (bacterial, fungal, protozoal, rickettsial and spirochaetal) causes have been described.

Myocardial biopsy is considered to be the gold standard but in-flammatory changes may be patchy and normal myocardium may be biopsied. In addition, interpretation of the biopsy is subjective and the procedure is not without risk with the thin myocardium of dilated cardiomyopathy/myocarditis. Other confusing factors for the physician are that dilated cardiomyopathy can, like myocarditis, improve sponta-neously and myocarditis can develop into dilated cardiomyopathy. Therefore it is probably wise to consider and manage patients with myocarditis similarly to those with dilated cardiomyopathy in terms of decision strategy.

MANAGEMENT

Angiotensin converting enzyme inhibitors are the principle group of drugs that prolong survival in adults with left ventricular dysfunction, and in children too they have become very important. Hypotension should be avoided, particularly in those children who have a high renin because of dehydration from pre-existing diuretic treatment. Usually, treatment is started at a low dose which is progressively increased. Blood pressure is usually measured every 15 minutes after a test dose of captopril, e.g. 0.1 mg/kg (less if dehydrated). The captopril dose is steadily increased up to 1–2 mg/kg/24 h (given in three divided doses).

Diuretics are useful in improving symptoms of congestive heart failure. Fluid restriction may be needed initially, particularly if there is hyponatraemia, which usually does not need treatment with extra salt.

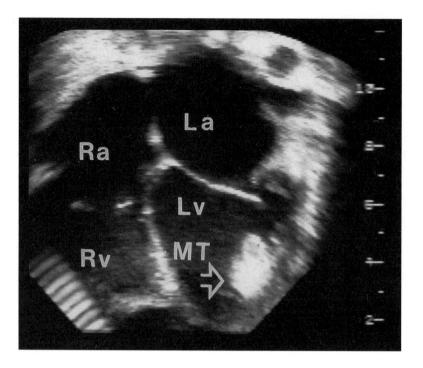

Figure 11.1   Cardiac ultrasound scan. Apical four-chamber view in dilated cardiomyopathy, showing a mural thrombus (MT) in the left ventricle (Lv). Ra = right atrium; La = left atrium; Rv = right ventricle.

Digoxin may have a positive inotropic effect, but its role remains unclear. Beta-blockers have been used in adults with dilated cardiomyopathy and have improved cardiac function, but they are not used widely in children. Occasionally, intravenous inotropes and vasodilators are needed. Dobutamine is a common first choice in this setting.

Anticoagulation is usually given to avoid embolization from intracavity thrombus (Figure 11.1). Heparin or warfarin is used when myocardial function is very poor, but this is usually changed to aspirin therapy alone in improving, more stable patients.

Arrhythmias should be treated if they are causing symptoms, but most anti-arrhythmic drugs are negatively inotropic and should be used with caution.

PROGNOSIS

Actuarial survival of dilated cardiomyopathy is around 60% at 5 years, although the outcome may be better in infants. When there is no improvement in systolic function, referral for cardiac transplantation may be necessary. Dilated cardiomyopathy is the commonest reason for cardiac transplantation in children and the outcome is better than that of transplantation for other heart diseases in children. Although actuarial survival after transplantation is in the region of 80% or higher at 3 years, the medium- and long-term future is uncertain. In general, transplantation is reserved for children who continue to deteriorate despite maximum medical therapy. The decision has to be made early as 50% of the deaths occur within 3 months of presentation and many children die awaiting a donor heart. This has led to the development of mechanical bridges to transplantation. These are popularly referred to as 'artificial hearts' and act as left ventricular assist devices, working from an external power source. Smaller, long-term implants are now available and it is likely that such devices may be used in paediatric practice in future.

Hypertrophic cardiomyopathy

Hypertrophic cardiomyopathy is based on the diagnosis of unexplained ventricular hypertrophy. Most children are asymptomatic on diagnosis. Often they have been referred with a murmur, which can sound remarkably innocent (particularly if there is no outflow obstruction), or they have been referred for family screening because a first-degree relative has the disease. Infants with hypertrophic cardiomyopathy are more likely to be symptomatic and present with cardiac failure.

PHYSICAL EXAMINATION

Physical signs vary with the severity of left ventricular outflow obstruction. The apex beat can have a double impulse. The pulse is fast-rising. The murmur is variable and can sound innocent, or resemble mitral regurgitation or aortic stenosis. Occasionally a mitral inflow murmur is audible. Obstruction is increased by the Valsalva manoeuvre and by standing.

CARDIAC INVESTIGATIONS

These include an ECG, which will show ventricular hypertrophy, often abnormal Q waves and abnormal ST segments or T waves. ECG abnormalities may precede echocardiographic changes. Echocardiography demonstrates ventricular hypertrophy which is typically asymmetrical (Figure 11.2).

Two-dimensional echo is better than M-mode because of the asymmetry. Occasionally, the hypertrophy can be purely apical. Often there is systolic anterior motion of the mitral valve, which contributes to left

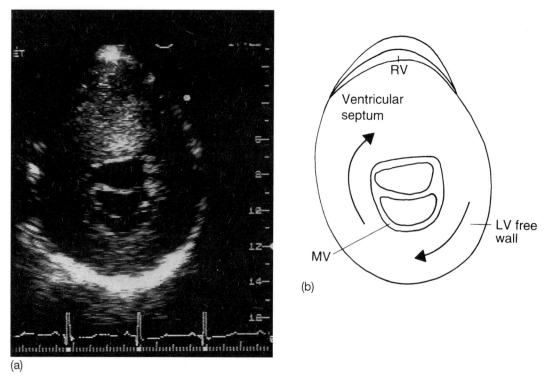

(a)

(b)

Figure 11.2   Cardiac ultrasound scan. (a) Short-axis view of severe hypertrophic cardiomyopathy. (b) Diagram of scan shown in (a) MV = mitral valve; RV = right ventricle.

ventricular outflow tract obstruction. Ambulatory electrocardiographic monitoring is usually undertaken, and it is generally assumed that there is an increased risk of sudden death if non-sustained ventricular tachycardia is detected, although this is probably only true in adults. Invasive electrophysiology testing has yet to be evaluated in young children, but it is used in adults to predict those at risk of sudden death.

NOONAN'S SYNDROME

Noonan's syndrome is an important cause of childhood hypertrophic cardiomyopathy: perhaps as many as one-third of all cases are linked to Noonan's syndrome. The myocardial disease is histologically similar to familial hypertrophic cardiomyopathy. Approximately 20% of Noonan's syndrome patients have cardiomyopathy. It can present in infancy, when it is usually associated with severe heart failure and these cases have a poor prognosis. When the cardiomyopathy is seen in later childhood, children are often asymptomatic. It is possible that sudden death is less common in Noonan's syndrome than in familial hypertrophic cardiomyopathy. Noonan's syndrome is an uncommon cause of adult hypertrophic cardiomyopathy: this may be because of the high attrition from cardiac failure in early life with Noonan's syndrome and cardiomyopathy, but may also be due to failure of recognition of the facial features, which become less marked with age.

INFANT HYPERTROPHIC CARDIOMYOPATHY

The major cause of ventricular hypertrophy in the newborn period is maternal diabetes, the increased fetal insulin acting as a growth factor. The prognosis is good, with spontaneous improvement occurring in infancy. In the most severe cases there can be heart failure and some deaths have been reported. Nesidioblastosis can also cause hypertrophy, for similar reasons, and other hyperinsulinaemic conditions include lipodystrophy, Beckwith–Wiedemann syndrome and Donohue's syndrome. It is quite possible that a number of cases of neonatal hypertrophic cardiomyopathy are caused by undiagnosed gestational diabetes and these may account for the patients with a cardiomyopathy who improve spontaneously. Neonatal dexamethasone treatment can induce hypertrophy, which resolves after treatment is stopped.

Usually, when children with hypertrophic cardiomyopathy develop heart failure in early infancy the prognosis is very poor with death occurring from progressive cardiac failure. A proportion of Noonan's syndrome patients present with heart failure in infancy as do some children with metabolic diseases (particularly Pompe's disease). A few cases of familial hypertrophic cardiomyopathy present in infancy, but for the idiopathic cases of hypertrophy that present with heart failure the prognosis is poor.

FAMILIAL HYPERTROPHIC CARDIOMYOPATHY

The term 'hypertrophic cardiomyopathy' is often used exclusively for this group of patients. In most cases inheritance is autosomal dominant, although there are a number of sporadic cases. Hypertrophy may often not develop until later childhood or puberty. The exact incidences are unknown because of varied clinical expression. Occasionally the first presentation can be sudden death. Indeed, sudden death is the principal cause of death from adolescence onwards, with a mortality of 2–6% of patients per year. Younger adolescent patients are at the highest risk of sudden death. Post-mortem reveals myocyte disarray.

TREATMENT

When there is associated left ventricular outflow tract obstruction, surgery can relieve symptoms, such as exercise induced syncope, or angina, but surgery may not alter the incidence of sudden death. Medical treatment with propranolol can also help symptoms related to both obstruction and to abnormal filling and verapamil may be helpful for the latter. Disopyramide may reduce the degree of obstruction, but should be used in conjunction with a beta-blocker because of potential rapid conduction of atrial arrhythmias.

Prevention of sudden death remains very difficult. A family history of sudden death is a very important prognostic risk factor, as (obviously) is survival of a cardiac arrest. It is apparent that some gene deletions are more malignant and ultimately risk may be stratified using molecular genetics. In patients at increased risk of sudden death it is possible that oral amiodarone therapy may be helpful, although there is some controversy about this as it has a proarrhythmic effect. Currently it is considered wise to advise children with familial hypertrophic cardio-myopathy to avoid competitive sport.

Treatment of infant symptomatic cardiomyopathy is with a beta-blocker such as propranolol, (occasionally verapamil is substituted) and diuretics. Very high dose propranolol is occasionally used. When heart failure is intractable transplantation is considered.

MOLECULAR GENETICS

There have been great advances in the molecular genetics of hyper-trophic cardiomyopathy recently. Restriction fragment length poly-morphic markers have localized the gene to chromosome 14 in a large French-Canadian family. Subsequently, a number of missense point mutations in the beta-myosin heavy-chain gene have been identified and, as discussed above, the risk of sudden death appears to vary with differing mutations.

Restrictive cardiomyopathy

Restrictive cardiomyopathy is rare in childhood. There may be some overlap with hypertrophic cardiomyopathy and it is clear that some cases of Noonan's syndrome can have a restrictive cardiomyopathy. In essence there is reduced ventricular compliance with normal systolic function and no ventricular hypertrophy.

A number of diseases are known to produce a secondary restrictive cardiomyopathy, but the most common causes in adults (amyloid, sarcoid and Fabry's disease) are virtually never seen in children. Pseu-doxanthoma elasticum is a very rare cause of restrictive cardiomyo-pathy.

Loeffler's disease is one of the hypereosinophilic syndromes and occurs sporadically throughout the world. There may be eosinophilic infiltration of organs other than the heart. A similar cardiac disease is seen when the eosinophilia is secondary to parasitic infection, drug reaction or polyarteritis nodosa. Pathologically there is fibrosis of the endocardium and the disease is commonly termed 'endomyocardial fibrosis'; this term is also used in idiopathic cases where there is no eosinophilia.

With restrictive cardiomyopathy, either the left or right ventricle can be involved with either mitral or tricuspid valve regurgitation. With right ventricular involvement there may be ascites and pericardial effusions. Although the ventricular cavities are normal or reduced, the atrial enlargement can result in cardiomegaly on the chest X-ray. Atrial arrhythmias are common and conduction disturbances have been reported. Embolic complications may also occur. It can be difficult to determine whether there is a restrictive cardiomyopathy or constrictive pericarditis. Typically, at cardiac catheterization there is a rise in atrial pressure with inspiration with the restrictive cardiomyopathy. Also, an increase in ventricular filling will cause varied elevation of ventricular diastolic pressures with cardiomyopathy. On echocardiography there are usually patchy bright echoes from the endocardium and the papillary muscles, the ventricles are small and the atria are dilated, whereas with constrictive pericarditis there may be obviously abnormal pericardium and calcification. When there is uncertainty it may be necessary to perform a pericardial biopsy and/or an endomyocardial biopsy.

The prognosis for restrictive cardiomyopathy is uncertain as there are very few children with the disease. In our experience many children remain quite well although when symptoms eventually develop they can deteriorate rapidly. They are also at increased risk for transplantation as there may be an elevation of the pulmonary vascular resistance, which can result in acute, severe heart failure post-transplant. Medical treatment is difficult as diuretics and vasodilators may severely reduce preload. Verapamil has been put forward as a possible treatment and steroids have been used in some cases of Loeffler's disease and eosinophilia syndromes.

Arrhythmogenic right ventricle

In this disease there is an abnormal area of dysplasia (fatty infiltration and fibrosis) in the right ventricular free wall, which can lead to ventricular arrhythmias. Symptoms tend to worsen with age and, although sudden death can occur, it is less common in children than in adults. The ventricular tachycardia and ventricular ectopics have a left bundle branch block pathology as they arise from the dysplastic areas. Some cases are familial and there have been advances in gene mapping recently. Uhl's anomaly may be a severe form of arrhythmogenic right ventricle with widespread right ventricular involvement, which can mirror the clinical presentation of Ebstein's disease

The ECG characteristically shows T wave inversion in leads V1–V4 in adults with arrhythmogenic right ventricle, but this finding is less specific in paediatrics. Signal averaging techniques for postexcitation waves in the ST segments are useful. Echocardiography can be normal in children, but may demonstrate abnormalities in the right ventricle, e.g. an outpouching, paradoxical motion of the free wall, or diffuse right ventricular dysfunction. Angiography may show dyskinesis and biopsy of the right ventricle can demonstrate the pathology. Treatment is initially with antiarrhythmic drugs, although occasionally surgical excision and/or catheter ablation have been used.

Secondary causes of heart muscle disease

PHYSICAL EXAMINATION

Physical examination can detect many secondary causes of hypertrophy. Hypertension is easily detected. The variety of diseases that have increased insulin levels often have marked dysmorphic features e.g. Beckwith–Wiedemann syndrome, generalized lipodystrophy and Donohue's syndrome. Thyroid disease and acromegaly may be obvious on physical examination. Dysmorphic features of Noonan's and leopard syndrome are usually apparent in children. Evidence of ataxia suggests Friedreich's disease. The mucopolysaccharidoses usually have typical clinical findings. Hepatosplenomegaly and central nervous system changes are seen with other lysosomal disease. GM_2-gangliosidosis may be associated with a cherry red macula. A skeletal myopathy is sometimes associated with a cardiomyopathy and is usually obvious. With Kearns–Sayre syndrome there is also external ophthalmoplegia. Cataracts are often associated with metabolic disease.

The investigations are detailed in Table 11.1. They are common to all cardiomyopathy cases, except where indicated.

CONNECTIVE TISSUE DISEASES

Connective tissue disorders such as SLE may develop a cardiomyopathy and some cases of congenital complete heart block (with maternal lupus or anti-Ro antibody) may progress to a dilated cardiomyopathy. This may be related to early autoimmune damage to the myocardium or progressive disease.

Table 11.1 Investigations for secondary heart muscle disease

- Physical examination (see text)
- Cardiac investigations (see text)
- Bloods
  - Autoimmune/connective tissue screen
  - Creatine kinase
  - Carnitine (free and acyl carnitine)
  - Fasting sugar and lactate
  - Thyroid function
  - Calcium/phosphate
  - Full blood count and film (eosinophilia or neutropenia)
  - Amino acids
  - Vacuolated lymphocytes
  - Possibly selenium (if geographical risk)
  - Iron and iron binding
- Urine
  - Amino acids
  - Organic acids
- Myocarditis investigations (usually taken in dilated cardiomyopathy too)
  - Serology for: Coxsackie, ECHO, influenza, parainfluenza, mumps, rubella and rubeola viruses and possibly HIV (non-viral causes should be considered)
  - Cardiac biopsy may be required
- Skeletal muscle biopsy
  - If skeletal myopathy suspected

Cardiac catheterization and angiography are not usually required, although it is sometimes necessary to exclude an anomalous coronary artery if echocardiography is unsatisfactory. Typically the ECG will demonstrate evidence of ischaemia.

SKELETAL MYOPATHIES

Muscular dystrophies and myopathies should also be considered. Duchenne's and Becker's muscular dystrophy will ultimately affect the myocardium (initially with hypertrophy but later with a progressive dilated cardiomyopathy) and recently it has been recognized that some families have X-linked cardiomyopathy with an abnormality of the dystrophin gene but no skeletal myopathy. These patients become symptomatic in adolescence and the cardiomyopathy is rapidly progressive. Creatinine kinase MM is elevated and therefore should be included as part of the screen for dilated cardiomyopathy.

Another X-linked condition is Barth's syndrome, which involves abnormal skeletal musculature, intermittent neutropenia and abnormal mitochondria.

Limb girdle muscular dystrophy may be associated with atrial arrhythmias and even atrial standstill. Other skeletal myopathies can involve the heart, e.g. juvenile progressive spinal muscular atrophy, Emery–Dreifuss dystrophy, facioscapulohumeral dystrophy, nemaline myopathy, myotubulin myopathy and the mitochondrial myopathies.

MITOCHONDRIAL MYOPATHIES

On skeletal muscle biopsy there may be unusual ragged-red fibres with trichrome staining, and the mitochondrial morphology is abnormal. A variety of enzyme deficiencies in the mitochondria have been described that produce both skeletal features and cardiomyopathy. There are also some patients who have the clinical and pathological features of a mitochondrial myopathy, but as yet no specific enzyme deficiency has been identified.

Carnitine is required to transport long-chain fatty acids across the mitochondrial membrane, and acyl-CoA dehydrogenase is important in beta-oxidation of fatty acids in the mitochondria; there are various types of the latter enzyme that deal with short-, medium- and long-chain fatty acids. Specific problems include primary carnitine deficiency, acyl-CoA dehydrogenase deficiency, electron transfer flavo protein (and dehydrogenase) deficiency and cytochrome c oxidase deficiency. Kearns–Sayre syndrome is a phenotype that consists of external ophthalmoplegia, pigmentary retinopathy and heart block.

In some of these conditions there may be non-ketotic hypoglycaemia, elevated ammonia and lactate, with an encephalopathy that can be fasting-related. The cardiomyopathy is usually hypertrophic with reduced systolic function but is occasionally dilated. When low plasma carnitine and acyl carnitine concentrations are found (i.e. low free and total carnitine) a primary carnitine deficiency is probable and these children often respond well to carnitine therapy. When the cardiomyopathy is due to a secondary carnitine deficiency (i.e. increased esterification of acyl-CoA to acyl carnitine with high plasma and urine concentrations of acyl carnitine) the cardiomyopathy may not respond to carnitine replacement therapy.

GLYCOGEN STORAGE DISEASES (GSD)

GSD-IIA is autosomal-recessive acid maltase deficiency (there is a type B that presents at an older age with a variable life expectancy). With type IIA (Pompe's disease) there is glycogen deposition in the heart, skeletal muscle and the liver. The ECG shows a short PR interval with increased ventricular voltages. Echocardiography demonstrates progressive, severe ventricular hypertrophy. Physical examination will usually reveal hepatomegaly and muscle weakness. Death usually occurs in early infancy from cardiorespiratory failure or aspiration from swallowing difficulties. Screening of the blood for vacuolated lymphocytes is helpful with GSD-II. Diagnosis can be confirmed using white blood cell enzyme assay although sometimes fibroblast culture or skeletal muscle biopsy are used. Prenatal diagnosis is now available by culturing cells obtained at amniocentesis.

Another glycogen storage disease with cardiac manifestations is GSD-III, which leads to hepatomegaly, fasting hypoglycaemia and skeletal myopathy. Although some degree of ventricular hypertrophy is common, severe hypertrophy will often not become manifest until later childhood or early adult life. GSD-IV may present in infancy or in later childhood with heart failure from a dilated cardiomyopathy.

MUCOPOLYSACCHARIDOSES AND MUCOLIPIDOSES

The mucopolysaccharidoses include MPS-I – Hurler's syndrome, autosomal recessive – and MPS-II – Hunter's syndrome, X-linked recessive. There is an accumulation of mucopolysaccharide in the valves, particularly the mitral and aortic valves, causing severe regurgitation and heart failure. There is also coronary artery narrowing, which can result in angina and infarction. The heart is dilated when there is severe heart failure but usually on echocardiography there is hypertrophy. The other forms of MPS cause less severe cardiac involvement, although occasionally a dilated cardiomyopathy is seen.

The mucolipidoses include I-cell disease, where the fibroblasts have multiple inclusions known as I cells. The heart typically has symmetrical hypertrophy and the valves may be involved.

GLYCOPROTEINOSES

Cardiac involvement has been reported in some of the glycoproteinoses, e.g. mannosidosis (short PR interval on ECG), fucosidosis and sialidosis (variable ventricular hypertrophy/dilatation).

LIPIDOSES

Cardiac involvement has also been reported in the lipidoses (for example Gaucher's disease with restrictive cardiomyopathy), multiple sulphatase deficiency (ventricular hypertrophy), Farber's disease (subcutaneous nodules, cardiomegaly and intracardiac nodules), and

Fabry's disease (the ventricular hypertrophy is uncommon in children).

GANGLIOSIDOSES

Both GM_1 and GM_2 gangliosidoses may be associated with myocardial hypertrophy/dilatation and left-sided valve involvement has been reported.

CARDIOTOXINS

A small number of cardiotoxins are recognized as causing dilated cardiomyopathy. There include iron (haemochromatosis), where the heart is often dilated and hypertrophied with reduced ventricular function and restriction to filling. It may be primary, although this rarely causes symptoms in childhood and secondary haemochromatosis, usually related to thalassaemia or other haematological disease, is more common. Copper (in Wilson's disease) can result in a dilated cardiomyopathy, as can lead. Alcoholic-dilated cardiomyopathy is not seen in children. Chloroquine and hydroxychloroquine may have a cardiotoxic effect.

The major group of cardiotoxins seen in paediatric practice are agents used in chemotherapy, principally anthracyclines but also cyclophosphamide and cis-platinum. Mediastinal irradiation can damage the myocardium and result in chronic pericardial disease. There has been much recent research on the effects of anthracycline on the heart; it can have both an acute and chronic effect. The incidence of late-onset congestive heart failure is related to the dose and possibly the speed of infusion: it is found in over 30% with doses of over 550 mg/m^2. Slow infusions may also reduce the toxicity. Irradiation to the thorax or upper abdomen increases the incidence of myocardial dysfunction.

OTHER CAUSES OF CARDIOMYOPATHY

Refsum's disease is a peroxisomal disorder with abnormal phytanic acid storage. The main findings are usually neurological, but a dilated cardiomyopathy associated with heart block has been reported. Other systemic diseases that should be considered are thyroid disease, hypocalcaemia, hypophosphataemia, chronic anaemia, malnutrition, beri-beri and selenium deficiency (also called Keshan disease as it is more common in this region of China, where the selenium-poor soil results in a deficiency of a cytoplasmic enzyme).

Acquired heart disease 12

In developed countries most cases of infective endocarditis in children occur in association with congenital heart disease. As expected, the most common lesions in clinical practice (bicuspid/stenotic aortic valves and unoperated VSDs) are the most common lesions involved in endocarditis.

It is clearly important to be explicit about the need for antibiotic prophylaxis for potential bacteraemic episodes when congenital heart disease has been diagnosed. The rather stark facts that infective endocarditis still has a mortality of around 20% and that the lifetime risk of endocarditis occurring in unoperated VSDs is probably in excess of 10%, reinforce this.

The greater the turbulence of flow around a lesion the higher the risk of infective endocarditis. This is because endothelial damage results in platelet and fibrin deposition, which can subsequently become infected. Therefore, the lesions at greatest risk include small VSDs, PDAs, mitral regurgitation, aortic regurgitation, severe outflow tract obstructions and aorto-pulmonary (Blalock) shunts. Prosthetic valves are also at greatly increased risk of developing endocarditis.

Although the likelihood of endocarditis is considerably reduced once a VSD is operated, at present this cannot justify the policy of operating on all small VSDs because of the risk of cardio-pulmonary bypass, but once a PDA has been diagnosed outside early infancy it is considered wise for the duct to be closed, as the risk of infective endocarditis is greater than the risk of surgical or transcatheter closure. Infective endocarditis is very rare in association with secundum ASDs (where there is a low pressure flow) and antibiotic prophylaxis is not required.

Infective endocarditis

CAUSATIVE ORGANISMS

Infective endocarditis has often been divided into acute and subacute, although it is probably more precise to define the disease by its causative organism and use the more broad term infective endocarditis.

The most common organisms are the *viridans* (alpha-haemolytic) streptococci. Infection is typically indolent, but some subspecies, e.g. *milleri*, give a more fulminant course, as do other streptococcal groups such as the pneumococci. However, most cases of fulminant infective endocarditis are caused by *Staphylococcus aureus* infection and, unlike the *viridans* infections, there may be no history of congenital heart disease. *Staphylococcus epidermidis* is increasingly recognized as a cause of endocarditis and typically is hospital acquired, occurring in immunosuppressed individuals, those with indwelling central lines and after cardiac surgery. The infection has a more indolent course than *Staphylococcus aureus* endocarditis.

Although other organisms causing infective endocarditis are well recognized, they are all uncommon. Candidal endocarditis has been documented in those patients who are also at risk of *Staphylococcus epidermidis* endocarditis. Large vegetations are common with candidal endocarditis and embolization is well documented. The prognosis is poor and late relapse can occur. Other infective organisms include anaerobes, Gram-negative (and occasionally Gram-positive) bacilli and Q fever.

PHYSICAL SIGNS

In most cases of endocarditis the onset is insidious, with general malaise, anorexia, arthralgia and a fever. The physical signs on examination will reflect the underlying congenital heart disease, although these can change, for example if valve regurgitation develops. Splenomegaly is common. The more classical signs of infective endocarditis (such as splinter haemorrhages, petechiae, haemorrhagic Janeway lesions, tender Osler's nodes on the extremities and retinal Roth's spots) are uncommon in childhood infective endocarditis.

LABORATORY INVESTIGATIONS

In most cases the causative organism is found in blood cultures but in at least 10% no organism is found. This number increases if recent antibiotics have been given, if the lesion is on the right (pulmonary side) of the heart or if an atypical organism such as *Candida* is the cause. Adequate volumes of blood must be taken using a strict aseptic technique with a proper skin preparation (not just an alcohol wipe), and usually six samples are taken from different sites in 24 hours in suspected infective endocarditis.

The ESR is elevated but is sometimes only mildly so when there is heart failure or renal failure. Rheumatoid factor and circulating immune complexes may be detected. The anaemia of chronic disease is found in approximately 50% of infective endocarditis in children. Although frank haematuria is uncommon, positive stick testing for microscopic haematuria occurs in virtually all cases of endocarditis.

ECHOCARDIOGRAPHY

This is helpful in establishing the diagnosis if vegetations (clusters of infected material consisting of fibrin and platelet deposition) are seen, but a negative echocardiogram does not exclude the diagnosis. When the vegetation is large there is an increased risk of embolization. Even with successful treatment a vegetation will be reabsorbed very slowly and a persistent echocardiographic abnormality should not increase the duration of treatment if there has been a successful response.

TREATMENT

Intravenous antibiotics are invariably used in the initial phase of treatment. The *viridans* streptococci are usually exquisitely sensitive to penicillin, so intravenous benzyl penicillin is used, in conjunction with low-dose intravenous gentamicin as this appears to be a good synergistic combination. The gentamicin is stopped after 2 weeks and oral amoxycillin is substituted for the intravenous penicillin at the same time. Antibiotics are then continued for a further 2 weeks. Some streptococci (e.g. *Streptococcus faecalis*) have a reduced sensitivity to penicillin, so low-dose gentamicin and intravenous penicillin are continued for at least 4 weeks.

Endocarditis caused by *Staphylococcus aureus* is treated with intravenous flucloxacillin and either gentamicin or fucidic acid for at least 4 weeks. Again, the gentamicin is usually stopped after 2 weeks. Rifampicin may be helpful in difficult cases.

In cases of penicillin allergy, vancomycin or teicoplanin are usually substituted and can be used as a single agent. Vancomycin is also used for *Staphylococcus epidermidis* and methicillin-resistant *Staphylococcus* infections. Rarer causes of endocarditis require individualized antibiotic regimes.

The success of therapy is monitored by clinical markers such as fever and laboratory markers such as ESR and blood cultures. Investigations to determine whether adequate antibiotic levels have been achieved vary with different laboratories and should be discussed with the local department. In general, the minimum inhibitory concentration is determined and bactericidal titres in the blood are checked regularly with back titrations.

SURGERY

This is usually reserved for those cases where there is severe heart failure from valve disruption and valve replacement is required. Failure to eradicate the organism is also an indication for surgery, as are embolization and the presence of a large or friable vegetation that is considered to be at risk of embolization. Surgery is more commonly undertaken in fungal lesions and where there is prosthetic material (particularly a prosthetic valve).

COMPLICATIONS

The main cause of death with infective endocarditis is severe heart failure (which is mainly from valve disruption).

With left-side lesions emboli can be cerebral or renal and with right-side lesions there may be recurrent pulmonary emboli. Cerebral haemorrhage can occur, with rupture of a mycotic aneurysm. Abscess formation is well recognized and has been reported in the spleen, brain, aortic root and lung. Cerebral abscess formation can have a wide range of neurological symptoms and signs and should be suspected when any neurological symptoms develop in a child with congenital heart disease. In those with cyanosis and a right-to-left shunt there is loss of lung filtration; an abscess can develop without antecedent endocarditis. An abscess can sometimes occur in children with left-sided endocarditis and subsequent embolization of vegetations. Aortic root abscess is usually catastrophic and induces rapidly progressive aortic regurgitation. The resulting very low diastolic pressure can sometimes be mistaken for bacteraemic/septic shock. Surgery is invariably required for an aortic root abscess and is high-risk.

Immune complex disease can occur and glomerulonephritis is occasionally seen.

PREVENTION

Good dental health should be encouraged. Antibiotic prophylaxis is required for transient bacteraemia in any child with congenital (except isolated ostium secundum or sinus venosus ASDs) or rheumatic heart disease (Table 12.1).

Cover should be given for all dental procedures. The *viridans* streptococci are common mouth and gastrointestinal flora. Surgical procedures should also be covered, as should deep lacerations that require suturing. Skin sepsis and infected eczema must be properly treated. The loss of

Table 12.1 Antibiotic prophylaxis

Oral treatment

Not penicillin-allergic, no recent penicillin	> 10 years 3 g oral amoxycillin 1 h preop (5–10 years, 1.5 g, < 5 years 750 mg)
Penicillin-allergic, or received more than a single dose of penicillin within last month	> 10 years 600 mg oral clindamycin 1 h preop (5–10 years 300 mg, < 5 years 150 mg)

Intravenous treatment (preferred for high risk patients)

Not penicillin-allergic, no recent penicillin	> 10 years 1 g IV amoxycillin at induction (5–10 years 500 mg, < 5 years 250 mg) then 500 mg oral amoxycillin 6 h postop (5–10 years 250 mg, < 5 years 125 mg)
If high risk (previous endocarditis or prosthetic valve) or genitourinary procedure	Add gentamicin 120 mg IV given at induction (2 mg/kg < 10 years)
Penicillin-allergic, or received more than a single dose of penicillin within last month	Vancomycin 1 g, over at least 100 min, prior to procedure then gentamicin 120 mg at induction or 15 min prior to procedure (< 10 years vancomycin 20 mg/kg, gentamicin 2 mg/kg)
	Alternatively: At induction: IV teicoplanin 400 mg (< 14 years 6 mg/kg) and IV gentamicin 120 mg (< 10 years 2 mg/kg)

- We currently advise antibiotic prophylaxis for all obstetric, gynaecological and gastrointestinal procedures, although others will only treat 'high risk' patients with prophylaxis for these procedures
- When clindamycin is used in multistage procedures it should not be repeated at intervals of less than 2 weeks
- For genitourinary procedures with a concurrent urine infection an appropriate antibiotic for the organism should be added

Modified from the recommendations of the Working Party of the British Society for Antimicrobial Chemotherapy

deciduous teeth does not need to be covered. Ear- and body-piercing are inadvisable.

Pericarditis

Purulent pericarditis is uncommon in children and is usually a secondary infection from another source, particularly of the lung. *Staphylococcus aureus*, *Haemophilus influenzae* and *Streptococcus pneumoniae* are the most common pathogens. It can occur after cardiac surgery, in which case it is usually staphylococcal. Primary purulent infections are recognized. Viral infections can lead to pericarditis, in particular the Coxsackie group, which also cause myocarditis.

Post-pericardotomy syndrome

This syndrome occurs during the convalescent period after cardiac surgery and rarely becomes manifest less than a week after surgery. There is a high fever with malaise and occasionally chest pain. Echocardiography reveals a pericardial effusion although it is important to recognize that pericardial effusions are common after cardiac surgery and the post-pericardotomy syndrome should probably not be diagnosed unless there is systemic upset. Treatment is with anti-inflammatory drugs and the pericardial fluid should be monitored carefully with echocardiography.

Occasionally, effusion can be large and signs of cardiac tamponade develop, venous pressure becomes elevated, there is hepatomegaly, pulse volume is small with marked paradox (i.e. the volume is reduced on inspiration) and heart sounds are very soft. The chest X-ray shows a large, globular heart without increasing pulmonary vascular markings. The ECG has low voltage complexes and most patients have elevation of ST segments with widespread T wave inversion.

If the child is haemodynamically compromised by the effusion then emergency drainage is required. This can be performed from a subcostal approach, just lateral to the xiphisternum at approximately 45% of cranio-caudal angulation and 45% of oblique angulation (which is virtually towards the left shoulder). An alternative approach is near the apex in approximately the mid-clavicular line in the fourth left interspace. Often it is possible to insert a plastic intravenous cannula. Most of the effusions are serous, so it is easy to assess when fluid has been successfully entered; the needle can be removed and the cannula advanced.

ECG monitoring during aspiration is helpful and some advocate attaching an electrode to the advancing needle. Certainly, echocardiographic control is very useful as the largest area of fluid can be identified and the needle can then be aimed at the point at which the fluid has been visualized with the ultrasound.

Often by changing the child's position it is possible to move the pericardial fluid, so for example sitting the child up will increase the amount of fluid anteriorly if a subcostal approach is used. (When the fluid is loculated and in a posterior position it will not be possible to aspirate it successfully). If the fluid continues to reaccumulate at a rapid rate it may be necessary to position a drain and a pleuro-pericardial window may be required so that the fluid will successfully drain into the pleural space and tamponade will not develop again.

If recurrent effusions develop following cardiac surgery the possibility of a chylous collection (pericardial or pleural) should be considered. Occasionally, chylous pericardial effusions are seen *de novo*. If a child has been on a normal diet the fluid is milky white, but if he or she has been on intravenous fluid it may be more difficult to make the diagnosis. Microscopy will reveal an excess of lymphocytes in the fluid and triglyceride analysis can also be undertaken.

Treatment of recurrent chylous effusions is with a low-fat diet with medium-chain triglyceride supplementation; alternatively, total parenteral nutrition can be used. Occasionally surgery is undertaken to try and identify the source of chylous leakage.

Rheumatic fever

Rheumatic fever is now uncommon in developed countries, with an incidence of 1–3/100 000 (and this typically represents mild disease), but the incidence rises to 1–2/1000 in developing countries and the disease is usually more severe. The changes in incidence are almost certainly related to improvements in social circumstances, one of the most important being the provision of adequate housing without overcrowding.

AETIOLOGY

The widespread use of antibiotics or a change in streptococcal virulence may also have had an effect on the reducing incidence because rheumatic fever is always associated with a concomitant streptococcal infection and this probably induces an abnormal immune response. Lancefield group A streptococci (*Streptococcus pyogenes*) are a subgroup of beta-haemolytic streptococci that account for most human streptococcal illnesses and the M-proteins on the cell wall are implicated in the abnormal immune response (possibly genetically determined) that induces rheumatic fever. Typically the disease begins after a sore throat and there may be a latent period of between 1 and 5 weeks although this is longer for Sydenham's chorea (2–6 months). Rheumatic fever is rare in infancy.

PATHOLOGY

Initially the changes are inflammatory, but subsequently there is proliferation with so called Aschoff's nodules and cells with typical 'owl-eye' nuclei. Acute rheumatic fever typically has a pancarditis with involvement of the pericardium, producing an effusion, of the myocardium, resulting in reduced contractility, and of the endocardium, affecting the valves and the chorda tendineae. The left-side valves are

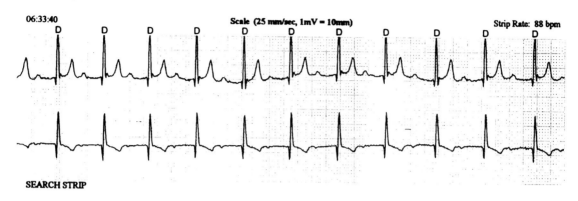

Figure 12.1 ECG (from ambulatory recording) showing prolonged PR interval (280 ms) in acute rheumatic fever.

principally affected and the mitral valve is more commonly affected than the aortic. Initially there is valve regurgitation, but eventually adhesions lead to valve stenosis. A severe early carditis is a poor prognostic marker and conversely if there is minimal initial carditis the subsequent valve disease is usually mild. Often the conduction tissue is involved in the carditis and typically this manifests itself with some degree of heart block, usually first-degree (Figure 12.1).

INVOLVEMENT OF OTHER SYSTEMS

A migratory polyarthritis of the large joints is seen with acute rheumatic fever; it does not lead to chronic changes. Dermatological changes include subcutaneous nodules and erythema marginatum; both are rare and are not pathognomonic (nodules are sometimes seen with rheumatoid arthritis and SLE; central clearing erythema is sometimes seen with drug reactions). Neurological involvement in rheumatic fever usually manifests itself as chorea (Sydenham's chorea or St Vitus' dance). The onset is insidious, with mild initial symptoms. The chorea tends to be self-limiting but it can be very severe. Haloperidol is given to relieve symptoms and benzodiazepines are also given to provide sedation.

DIAGNOSIS

The diagnosis is based on the modified Jones criteria (Table 12.2). The Jones criteria are not ideal and can lead to both over- and under-diagnosis. Unfortunately there is no specific test.

Table 12.2 Modified Jones criteria

Major criteria	*Minor criteria*
Arthritis, carditis, chorea, erythema marginatum, subcutaneous nodules	Fever, arthralgia, elevated acute phase reactants (ESR or CRP), first degree heart block, previous history of rheumatic fever

Rheumatic fever is diagnosed if two major or one major and two minor criteria are present in addition to evidence of recent streptococcal infection – raised ASO titre, positive throat swab or recent scarlet fever

The antistreptolysin O antibody (ASO titre) is over 500 units in most cases of acute rheumatic fever, declining to normal over 6 months. When it is borderline, alternative antistreptococcal antibodies should be assessed, e.g. antideoxyribonuclease-B and antistreptokinase.

TREATMENT

The most important treatment is preventative and if socioeconomic conditions can be improved in developing countries it seems inevitable that the incidence of rheumatic fever will fall. In acute rheumatic fever the treatment involves initial eradication of any streptococcal infection with penicillin and also anti-inflammatory treatment. Aspirin is given in divided doses of up to 120 mg/kg/d. Serum salicylate levels should be monitored. Usually, the full dose is continued for 2 weeks and then reduced to half of the initial dose. Once evidence of inflammation has disappeared, judged by clinical and laboratory markers (which may take a month or more), the aspirin is gradually tailed off.

Corticosteroids tend to be reserved for when there is evidence of acute carditis. They have a more rapid effect than aspirin and probably decrease the carditis more quickly, although there is no firm evidence that they reduce the risk of cardiac damage.

Heart failure requires treatment in the usual ways (pp. 73–5) until valvar regurgitation has improved. Urgent valve replacement is sometimes required. Heart block very rarely requires treatment.

Prophylaxis with antibiotics is given on a long-term basis. Certainly it is continued throughout childhood and in some countries is continued for life. This is to prevent recurrences, and seems to significantly reduce the risk of subsequent valvular heart disease. Penicillin is given either as a monthly intramuscular injection or as a twice a day oral preparation. Erythromycin is used if there is penicillin allergy.

Connective tissue disease

JUVENILE RHEUMATOID ARTHRITIS AND SYSTEMIC LUPUS ERYTHEMATOSUS

Pericarditis is the most common cardiac manifestation of both juvenile rheumatoid arthritis (JRA) and SLE (particularly drug-induced). It is usually mild and, although drainage is occasionally undertaken to exclude a purulent infection, it is uncommon for therapeutic aspiration to be needed. In both conditions non-steroidal anti-inflammatory drugs are used for mild cases and steroids for more severe ones. In JRA pericarditis can precede the onset of arthritis, although it usually develops months or even years afterwards and is more common in systemic onset JRA during a recrudescence of symptoms.

Myocarditis is less common in both JRA and SLE. When it does occur, anti-failure treatment may be necessary. With SLE there may be involvement of conduction tissue, which can cause heart block or arrhythmias. Valve involvement is even more rare, but it has been documented in both diseases and principally affects the aortic valve. Libman and Sacks described sterile vegetations in SLE and rheumatoid nodules have been documented on valves in JRA although they are usually too small to be seen on echo. Myocardial infarction is another rare complication of SLE and it is probably linked to the presence of lupus anticoagulant (a misnomer) and antibody to cardiolipin (neither of which are specific to SLE) and/or an arteritis. Hypertension can be a severe problem with SLE.

The cardiac manifestations of neonatal lupus are described in Chapter 5. Children with congenital complete block secondary to maternal SLE/anti-Ro antibody do appear to be at risk of developing dilated cardiomyopathy in later childhood.

SPONDYLO-ARTHROPATHIES

Aortic insufficiency is well documented, particularly with ankylosing spondylitis although it is uncommon in children. Occasionally it can precede sacro-ileitis. Conduction defects are also seen, but again are more common in adults.

Kawasaki's disease

Kawasaki first described this disease in 1967 and the annual incidence in Japan (where it is most common) is estimated at 100/100 000 preschool children, although it is 9/100 000 in the USA and less (1–3/100 000) in the UK. There is a slight preponderance of males and the mortality is also worse in males. Kawasaki's disease is uncommon in school-age children, rare over the age of 10 and uncommon in neonates. The aetiology is unknown, although an infective precipitant has been postulated as there have been a few clusters of cases and occasionally recurrent disease is seen.

DIAGNOSTIC CRITERIA FOR KAWASAKI'S DISEASE

- Fever of 5 or more days.
- Presence of four of the five conditions below:
  - bilateral conjunctival injection;
  - changes in the mucosa of the oropharynx (i.e. strawberry tongue, dry cracked lips, injected pharynx);
  - changes in the extremities (e.g. oedema, erythema, desquamation which usually occurs after the first week of illness; Plate 2);
  - polymorphous rash;
  - a cervical lymphadenopathy.

DIFFERENTIAL DIAGNOSIS

This should include staphylococcal and streptococcal infections (notably scarlet fever), Stevens–Johnson syndrome, drug reactions, juvenile rheumatoid arthritis, mycoplasma, viral exanthems, rickettsial disease and leptospirosis. With Kawasaki's disease the peeling tends to be limited to the hands and feet, unlike scarlet fever (where it is generalized desquamation, with no conjunctival congestion and it usually occurs in older children).

Other features of Kawasaki's disease are:

- reddening and crust formation at the site of previous BCG (often more marked after infant inoculation);
- arthralgia/arthritis;
- extreme irritability and sometimes aseptic meningitis;
- hepatic dysfunction and there may be hydrops of the gall bladder;
- diarrhoea;
- pneumonitis;
- otitis media;
- uveitis;
- urethritis.
- thrombocytosis (usually occurs after the first week).

CARDIAC PROBLEMS

The mortality rate in Kawasaki's disease is 0.5–2% and is principally from myocardial infarction. In the initial phase there may be a gallop rhythm. The ECG can show PR and QT prolongation and ST segments may be altered. Arrhythmias are rare. Myocarditis and pericarditis are

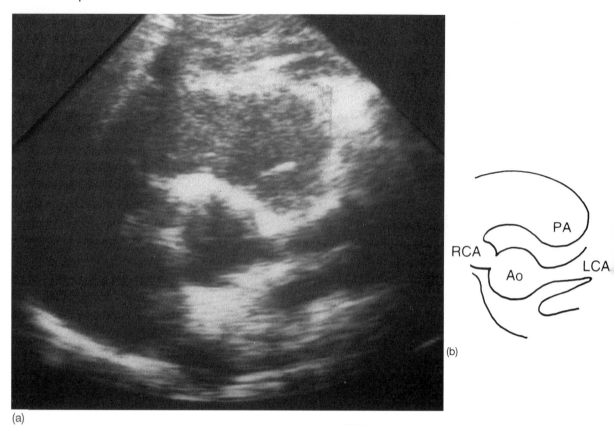

(a)

(b)

sometimes seen on echocardiography, with valvar regurgitation, reduced contractility and pericardial fluid. There is characteristic coronary involvement from vasculitis (which can affect other arteries). On
echocardiography, some dilatation of the proximal coronaries is common in the second week of the illness.

Aneurysms develop in around 20% of untreated children; half of
these will resolve over 2 years. The late development of aneurysms (> 3
months from the onset of the illness) is uncommon. Most deaths occur
within 3 months of the onset and are usually from myocardial infarction, although occasional deaths from acute myocarditis or rupture of
an aneurysm causing haemopericardium have been reported.

Echocardiography can visualize the proximal coronary arteries and if
enlarged they may be traced further. Distal disease is uncommon in the
absence of proximal abnormalities and probably more than 90% of
aneurysms are detected with echocardiography (Figure 12.2(a)).

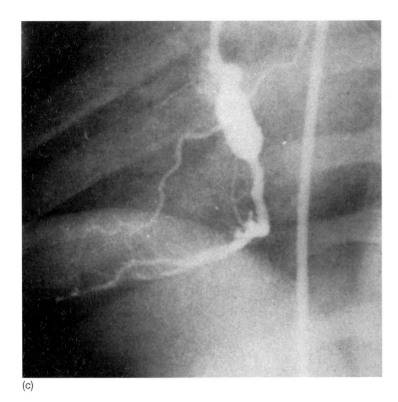

(c)

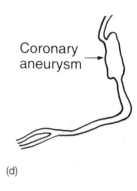

Coronary aneurysm →

(d)

Figure 12.2   Kawasaki disease. (a) Cardiac ultrasound scan. Parasternal short-axis view showing dilatation of left main coronary artery. (b) Diagram of scan shown in (a). (c) Angiogram of right coronary artery, showing giant aneurysm. (d) Diagram of features shown in (c). Ao = aorta; PA = pulmonary artery; RCA = right coronary artery; LCA = dilated left coronary artery. (a and c by kind permission of Dr I. Östman-Smith)

Occasionally resolution of the vasculitis results in coronary stenosis, which can lead to symptoms from myocardial ischaemia. It appears that coronary involvement is more likely when there has been a prolonged fever, or if there is peri/myocarditis. Occasionally giant coronary aneurysms (over 8 mm) are seen (Figure 12.2(c)) and these children are at high risk for myocardial infarction.

Echocardiography is usually performed when the clinical diagnosis is suspected and then approximately 2 weeks later, a third scan is performed one month after this. Further scans are sometimes performed at 3 months and 1 year follow up. When abnormalities are seen, echocardiography is repeated regularly until there is resolution. Exercise testing is occasionally helpful at longer-term follow-up for children who have had coronary involvement. Cardiac surgery and coronary grafting is very rarely required and is reserved for those cases with significant persistent cardiac symptoms.

TREATMENT

- **Initial**:
  - High-dose aspirin (30 mg/kg/d in three divided doses) until afebrile for 2 days.
  - Intravenous gammaglobulin 2 g/kg as a slow infusion over 8–12 h – effective if given within 10 days of the onset of symptoms (this will interfere with subsequent MMR vaccine, which should be delayed for at least 6 months).
- **Subsequent** (after the 14th day of illness in an afebrile child):
  - Aspirin 3–5 mg/kg/d once a day for 6–8 weeks unless there are proven coronary abnormalities (when continued until coronaries have returned to normal).
- **Acute myocardial infarction**:
  - Fibrinolytic therapy, e.g. streptokinase.

By using aspirin and immunoglobulin symptomatic inflammation is reduced and the risk of aneurysm development is significantly lower. Unfortunately it is sometimes difficult to make the diagnosis. Many of the diagnostic criteria are not uncommon in childhood illnesses and the disease can be both over- and underdiagnosed. The decision to treat atypical cases has to be made on an individual basis by an experienced clinician. Kawasaki's disease can be very difficult to diagnose in young infants.

Hypertension   Measurement of blood pressure is discussed on pp. 11–13 and normal blood pressures are given in Table 1.6, p. 12.

The difficulties of measuring blood pressure and problems with acceptable normal values make precise definition of hypertension difficult. There are a number of normal value charts available, all open to various criticisms, but the figures in Table 1.6 are derived from the American task force on hypertension in childhood and may be used to define hypertension as either a systolic or diastolic value above the 95th centile for age. Borderline hypertension exists if values between the 90th and the 95th centile are found. It is always assumed that attention has been paid to careful measurement with the child at rest and that values have been confirmed on several occasions, separated by some weeks or months in asymptomatic mild hypertension.

Table 12.3 Causes of hypertension

Group	Comment
Essential	Family history important
	Common in adolescents
	Rare in young children
Renal parenchymal disease	Any type
Renovascular disease	Artery stenosis/emboli/arteritis
	Vein thrombosis
Cardiovascular	Coarctation
	Large pulse volume (patent ductus arteriosus, aortic regurgitation)
Endocrine	Excess catecholamines, steroids or thyroxine
Neurological	Raised intracranial pressure
	Autonomic dysfunction
Drugs	Including steroids, cyclosporin

AETIOLOGY

Cardiovascular causes of hypertension are rarely found; coarctation of the aorta is the principal lesion to be diagnosed or excluded. Abnormalities of the abdominal aorta (middle aortic syndrome) are very rare and the systolic hypertension identified in occasional cases of aortic regurgitation and patent ductus arteriosus are easily recognized and are associated with low diastolic pressures, i.e. a large pulse volume. A brief outline of the causes of hypertension is given in Table 12.3. More detailed consideration of the subject of hypertension should be sought in general paediatric or paediatric renal disease texts.

INVESTIGATIONS

History and examination often allows many causes to be excluded. In practice, if a cardiac cause is not apparent clinically, a renal cause is sought. Detailed investigation and management of non-cardiac causes is outside the scope of this text.

Mild hypertension in the second decade is often essential and requires no more evaluation than clinical assessment, urine analysis, microscopy and culture, blood haematology, urea and creatinine estimation and a renal ultrasound examination. Younger children, those with severe hypertension and those with clinical clues of an underlying cause require detailed appropriate investigation.

Mild hypertension exists if values above the 95th centile are found, severe hypertension exists if values more than 8 mmHg above the 95th centile are found or if asymptomatic clinical evidence or target organ damage is detected, such as:

- **eyes:** retinal changes;
- **heart:** left ventricular hypertrophy (clinical, ECG, echocardiogram);
- **kidney:** proteinuria, haematuria.

Symptomatic hypertension (heart failure, neurological symptoms or signs) requires emergency investigation and treatment.

TREATMENT

Mild essential hypertension indicates the need for lifestyle advice (weight loss if relevant, healthy eating, exercise encouraged) and occasional follow-up. Severe essential hypertension usually warrants drug therapy in addition unless severe obesity exists, in which case diet alone may be tried initially. However, careful long-term follow-up of risks and benefits of drug therapy for essential hypertension in adolescence does not yet prove the value of treatment. Symptomatic hypertension must be treated. Secondary hypertension requires appropriate therapy for the

Table 12.4   Drug treatment of hypertension

Drug	Dose/route	Comment
Chlorothiazide	5 mg/kg orally 8-hourly	Initial drug Watch electrolytes
Propranolol	1–2 mg/kg orally 8-hourly	Add to or substitute for diuretic Not used in asthma
Atenolol	1–2 mg/kg orally once daily	Helps compliance
Metoprolol	1–2 mg/kg orally 8-hourly	β_1-selective: less likely to precipitate asthma
Captopril	0.3–0.6 mg/kg orally 8-hourly	Start with small dose, 0.1 mg/kg or less Watch for exaggerated fall in blood pressure; may cause hyperkalaemia and elevation of urea and creatinine; in which case dose needs reducing, also if troublesome cough caused

For urgent treatment, consider

Frusemide	1 mg/kg IV 4–6-hourly	
Labetalol	Infusion IV 1–3 mg/kg/h	
Phentolamine	Infusion IV 1–5 µg/kg/h	
Nifedipine	0.25–0.5 mg/kg orally	Repeat if necessary

underlying cause and usually drug treatment for blood pressure. Drug therapy involves building up treatment until satisfactory control is achieved (Table 12.4). There is a wide selection of possible agents, it is better to be familiar with just a small number.

Tropical medicine and paediatric cardiology

It would be wrong to overemphasize the importance of tropical diseases in cardiology practice. In tropical countries congenital heart disease, rheumatic fever and cardiomyopathy account for most of the workload for paediatric cardiologists. Some tropical diseases, however, do have cardiovascular effects, notably schistosomiasis and trypanosomiasis.

SCHISTOSOMIASIS

The eggs of the trematode worm migrate in the human body and may cause cardiovascular symptoms, chiefly from pulmonary hypertension though occasionally myocarditis may occur.

TRYPANOSOMIASIS

The American type of trypanosomiasis (Chagas' disease) is transmitted by insect bites and there is an acute, toxic stage of the illness that commonly includes a myocarditis. Subsequently there is a chronic disease with parasympathetic damage, resulting in gastrointestinal lesions and, in approximately half of infected cases, cardiomyopathy. Conduction disturbance is common.

The African form of trypanosomiasis is also insect-transmitted (by the tsetse fly) and can result in the so called African sleeping sicknesses. Myocarditis has been reported but conduction disturbances are less common than with Chagas' disease.

MALARIA

Malarial disease may involve the heart, but this is rarely severe enough to cause heart failure; more typically there are conduction changes on the ECG.

ENDOMYOCARDIAL FIBROSIS

This has been discussed in the cardiomyopathy section. It has been speculated that the constrictive endomyocardial fibrosis seen in Africa may be secondary to a parasitic infection.

TUBERCULOUS PERICARDITIS

Direct (from mediastinal nodes) or haematogenous spread may occur. Presentation is usually insidious but can be acute, with tamponade. Diagnosis can be difficult as in more than 50% there are no acid-fast bacilli in the fluid, but the Mantoux test is usually positive. Pericardial biopsy may be necessary. Constrictive pericarditis develops in approximately one-third of patients.

The young adult with congenital heart disease 13

An increasing number of children with complex congenital heart disease survive to adult life. As with other chronic diseases the hand-over of care between paediatrician and adult physician is a crucial time for patients and their families. The role of combined specialist clinics is important and paediatricians are likely to have a major input into the care of children with congenital heart disease during the second decade of life. During this period a clear plan needs to be made not only about the longer-term cardiac care but also about other medical and social issues.

Sports

This is covered in Chapter 10 (pp. 95–7).

Social issues

Sensible advice about the risk of social drugs should be incorporated into the adolescent clinic. Cigarette smoking should be discouraged and is potentially very dangerous in children with complex congenital heart disease, particularly in those with low flow pulmonary circulation (Fontan procedure). Alcohol should be discussed and the need to avoid alcoholic binges should be reinforced, particularly in anticoagulated patients. The possibility of young adults using illegal drugs should also be considered and addressed. The risk of endocarditis from intravenous drug abuse should be made clear as should the risk from water overload, which can occur in association with Ecstasy ingestion, as well as the danger of Ecstasy itself. Amphetamines are currently fashionable with teenagers but their arrhythmogenic effect is a potential problem for those with congenital heart disease.

For more severely affected young people there should be comprehensive information on social services and charitable support. For example, mobility allowances are enormously helpful. Local authorities often need supportive documentation if rehousing is considered. A number of charities offer holiday funds and there are additional supplementary charity funds, e.g. the Rowntree family fund. The possibility of home tuition should be addressed for those who are unable to cope with the rigours of schooling.

Decisions on careers are made during the second decade of life, but unfortunately careers officers at school may have limited experience of children with congenital heart disease and inappropriate advice is sometimes given. It does seem wise to advise adolescent patients to contact their paediatric cardiologist if there is difficulty regarding careers counselling, and this should help to prevent unfair discrimination during job applications. Similarly, there may need to be medical input into mortgage and life insurance applications, as insurers are rather cautious, because of the limited amount of long-term follow-up for some of the more complex congenital heart surgery that has been performed in the last 20 years.

Patient support groups are very helpful in all stages of care for patients with congenital heart disease. (In the UK there is a 'Grown-up Congenital Heart Disease Association'.)

Contraception and pregnancy

It is important that physicians begin discussions about contraception and pregnancy at an early stage of adolescence, as it is clear that the age at which sexual activity begins has decreased in the last few decades. In some conditions pregnancy can be very high-risk, notably in Eisenmenger's syndrome, and some would consider this to be an absolute contraindication to pregnancy. Other conditions with some increased maternal risk include young women with a Fontan circulation, cyanotic heart disease, severe outflow obstruction and Marfan's disease with a dilated ascending aorta, although successful pregnancies have been reported in these groups. There is also an increased risk of fetal loss with the Fontan circulation and cyanotic congenital heart disease, particularly if the oxygen saturation is below 85% (when there is a 50% risk of fetal death).

Patients should be made aware of the risk of recurrence of congenital heart disease in their offspring (Chapter 3). They should also be made aware of the availability of prenatal diagnosis using fetal echocardiography.

Oestrogen-containing oral contraceptives are contraindicated in cyanotic congenital heart disease, Eisenmenger's syndrome and the Fontan circulation because of the risk of thrombosis. The progesterone-only pill is an alternative, although it is less reliable. Intrauterine contraceptive devices are associated with an increased risk of endocarditis and are probably best avoided. Barrier methods of contraception are safe, but are not completely reliable. Therefore in high-risk young women, principally those with Eisenmenger's syndrome, the possibility of laparoscopic tubal ligation should be considered as a method of contraception unless there is a stable relationship and the male partner is prepared to have a vasectomy.

This has been dealt with in Chapter 12. General endocarditis prophylaxis advice should be given regularly, but it is important to reinforce the risk of activities such as ear- and other body-part-piercing, tattooing and intravenous drug abuse. **Infective endocarditis**

Patients with congenital heart disease are usually able to travel by air, although it is wise for the families to adequately inform the airlines of any problem. Often supplementary oxygen will be needed for children with significant cyanosis, heart failure or pulmonary hypertension. **Travel**

Many young adults with congenital heart disease seek a driving licence and in general only syncope precludes a standard driving licence. Certainly it is helpful for many young adults to hold a driving licence as this gives them an increased mobility.

Polycythaemia is related to the severity of cyanosis. Traditionally, the packed cell volume and haemoglobin are monitored and elective venesection is undertaken to prevent thromboembolic events. Recently there has been a tendency to delay venesection unless symptoms such as headache and paraesthesia develop, as frequent venesection can result in a more rapid rise in the haemoglobin and a complicating iron-deficiency anaemia. Microcytosis is a risk factor for cerebrovascular accident because of its effect on red cell deformity. If a venesection is performed it must be undertaken very slowly and an adequate fluid replacement given so that dehydration is avoided. If microcytosis/iron deficiency develop, iron should be given. **Polycythaemia**

Arrhythmias are often a complication of surgery, particularly when there has been extensive atrial surgery, e.g. in the early venous redirections undertaken for transposition (Mustard and Senning operation) and also after the Fontan operation, in which there is atrial distension. Arrhythmias are also seen following Fallot's tetralogy repair and for all of these conditions arrhythmia surveillance with an annual 24-hour ambulatory ECG is quite common. Whether the arrhythmias detected on ambulatory monitoring are markers of sudden death remains controversial and risk factor stratification for late sudden death following surgery for complex congenital heart disease continues to be modified. Symptomatic arrhythmias always require treatment. Bradyarrhythmias, particularly heart block, can develop after most intracardiac repairs and **Arrhythmias** for this reason adolescent clinics should include ECG analysis. Pacing is occasionally required.

Eisenmenger's syndrome

Eisenmenger's syndrome was described first in 1897. Essentially the lesion is that of progressive pulmonary vascular disease related to a left-to-right shunt, which, with high pulmonary flow and pressure, results in an increasingly elevated pulmonary vascular resistance to a level greater than the systemic vascular resistance, with eventual shunt reversal and cyanosis. The larger the lesion the greater the risk of pulmonary vascular disease developing. There is also an increased risk in children with Down's syndrome, probably because of the upper airway obstruction, which leads to hypoxia. Eisenmenger's disease will occur before the age of 1 year in children with Down's syndrome and atrioventricular septal defects.

As there has been a tendency towards earlier operation for congenital heart disease, there are far fewer with Eisenmenger's complex and the majority are now in adolescent and adult clinics rather than paediatric clinics. Surgical closure of the defect is not possible when shunt reversal has occurred as it would result in right ventricular failure.

Sudden death is well recognized and can be related to an arrhythmia or haemoptysis (as in the original case described by Eisenmenger). Haemoptysis is usually related to pulmonary artery thrombosis or bleeding from angiomas, which tend to develop in the pulmonary arteries. More commonly, death is from progressive heart failure, although death from endocarditis and cerebral abscess is also well recognized. Pregnancy and contraception are discussed above.

Surgery in adolescents and young adults

Re-operations are the principle problems for young adults with congenital heart disease. Occasionally an initial operation is performed in later childhood, for example when congenital heart disease was not detected earlier in life (as occasionally seen with ASDs) or if a lesion is becoming progressively more severe (such as aortic or mitral regurgitation, or aortic root dilatation in Marfan's syndrome). Re-operations may be needed if conduits or prosthetic valves become too small because of patient growth, or if they degenerate. Sometimes, obstruction can develop at anastomotic sites.

Re-operation in congenital heart disease is often technically very difficult. Even re-entry into the chest can be very demanding, particularly if there is a conduit in close proximity to the sternum. Increasingly, interventional cardiac catheterization is being undertaken in young adults. A common indication would be pulmonary artery stenosis related to previous cardiac surgery, and balloon dilatation, possibly with stent implantation, is probably preferable to re-operation. Balloon dilatation of the venous pathways in children who have had Mustard and Senning operations is occasionally required.

These are similar to those undertaken in the paediatric cardiology clinic. A 12-lead ECG is a helpful investigation to ensure that there is sinus rhythm and no evidence of heart block, also that voltages are not increasing and there is no evidence of ventricular strain. As discussed above, ambulatory monitoring is helpful to monitor for loss of sinus rhythm, bradycardias or pauses (which may require pacing) or asymptomatic atrial or ventricular arrhythmias. The merits of treating asymptomatic problems found on ambulatory monitoring are controversial (and should be discussed with the patient's individual cardiologist).

Regular investigations

ECHOCARDIOGRAPHY

As with young children this is a very useful investigation, but transthoracic pictures become more difficult to obtain in adolescents because of poor ultrasound penetration. Transoesophageal echocardiography is often undertaken to visualize the anatomy, but unfortunately is badly tolerated in this age group, even with heavy intravenous sedation, and general anaesthesia is often required. The latter is not without risk in young adults with congenital heart disease, particularly if there is evidence of severe outflow tract obstruction or pulmonary hypertension; vasodilatation and dehydration should be avoided with general anaesthesia.

LABORATORY INVESTIGATIONS

As discussed above (p. 133), haemoglobin and haematocrit are checked regularly in patients with cyanotic congenital heart disease. An absolute value at which venesection should be undertaken is difficult to establish as there is an increasing tendency to manage these patients conservatively, but a PCV of 65 or over probably represents a significant risk of cerebrovascular accident. Electrolytes are checked regularly in patients on diuretics and those taking angiotensin converting inhibitors, who will also need liver function tests and neutrophil counts. Plasma protein levels should be monitored in young adults with very high venous pressures particularly the Fontan type circuit, urine should be regularly stick-tested for proteinuria and the possibility of protein loss into the gut should be considered. Anticoagulation should be managed in appropriate local clinics as frequent blood testing is required.

EXERCISE TESTING

This is very difficult in early childhood but is much more practical in the second decade. Usually a modified Bruce protocol is used, but in more limited patients a flat walk over a set time (e.g. 12 minutes) is helpful to monitor progress.

Part Four
Arrhythmias

Arrhythmias 14

M. Runciman

There are a number of normal variations in heart rhythm, which need to be distinguished from pathological rhythm disturbances. The presence of an abnormal rhythm is not necessarily an indication for treatment. Identifying an arrhythmia as the cause for symptoms can be very difficult. An algorithm for the identification of cardiac rhythms from an ECG is given in Figure 14.1.

Introduction

These must be recognized to avoid unnecessary investigation and allow appropriate reassurance. Sinus rhythm is when impulses arise in the sinus node and are conducted through the atria and ventricles. Sinus rhythm is recognized on an ECG by P waves with a frontal axis of 0°–90° occurring before every QRS complex. Sinus arrhythmia (an increase in heart rate on inspiration) is normal and occurs in all children. The incidence of Wenckebach-type second degree heart block increases with age from 0% in neonates up to 15% in adolescents and is most evident when asleep. Heart rates in the 20s with pauses of up 4.5 s during sleep have been reported in otherwise healthy adolescent boys. Premature atrial contractions are common and seen in all age groups, including the fetus, while premature ventricular contractions are most commonly seen in the immediate neonatal period and in teenage years. Older children and adults can be aware of these premature contractions.

Normal rhythms

The presentation of clinically significant arrhythmias depends on the age of the child not only because certain arrhythmias are more common in certain age groups but also because the ability of children to tolerate arrhythmias, as well as their descriptive powers, changes with increasing age.

Presentation of abnormal rhythm

FETUS

Increasingly, fetal arrhythmias are being recognized, diagnosed and treated (pp. 64–5).

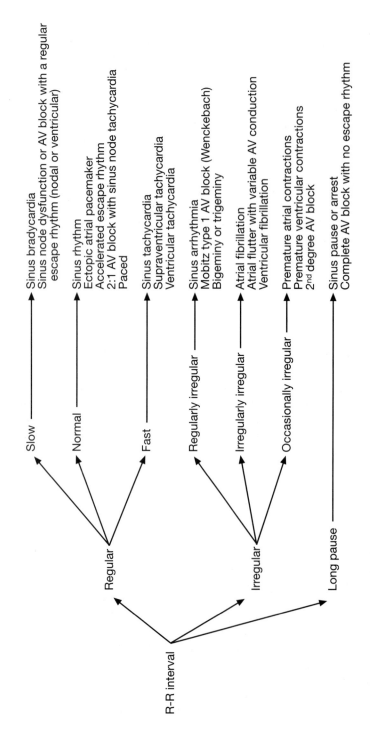

Figure 14.1 **Algorithm for the identification of cardiac rhythms** (derived from Park, M. K. and Guntheroth, W. G. (1992) *How to Read Pediatric ECGs*, 3rd edn, Year Book, Chicago, IL).

INFANCY

Arrhythmias in infancy are usually detected either by chance or because of heart failure. Transient bradycardias in this group are frequent during any intercurrent illness and are often secondary to respiratory irregularity or apnoea. The most commonly encountered primary arrhythmia in this group is SVT, which can rapidly lead to cardiac decompensation. It is important to differentiate SVT from an appropriate sinus tachycardia in an infant that is sick from another cause.

Sudden infant death syndrome (SIDS) remains the commonest cause of death in infants outside the neonatal period. Despite the well documented drop in incidence following advice on sleeping positions, temperature and smoking it still affects approximately 2/1000 infants. By definition there is no recognized cause and it is unknown whether or not some of these deaths are caused by arrhythmia.

CHILDHOOD

Presentation is usually with one of the following symptoms.

Irregular pulse is a frequent observation, and usually benign. It is normally caused by premature atrial or ventricular contractions.

Palpitations are a perceived abnormality of the heart rhythm. This is the commonest presenting feature of arrhythmias in children. The most frequent diagnosis will be supraventricular tachycardias, although ventricular tachycardias may have similar symptoms. Cardiac pain is uncommon in children, but occasionally they complain of this during palpitations.

Syncope is said to affect up to 15% of all children at some point. There are a number of causes (Table 14.1), although vasovagal syncope is the commonest.

It is usually possible to differentiate the causes if a careful history is taken from both the patient and an observer. Examination and an ECG is usually sufficient to diagnose the structural abnormalities likely to lead to syncope. Profound bradycardia or asystole are the commonest arrhythmias to cause cardiac syncope but ventricular tachycardia, whether associated with a prolonged QT syndrome or not, enter the differential. Tilt testing may be a valuable tool in detecting and evaluating autonomic dysfunction, although data from normal children is currently incomplete.

Heart failure is rarely the presenting feature of an arrhythmia in childhood. If it is, then an incessant tachycardia is the most likely cause and can be hard to distinguish from dilated cardiomyopathy.

Table 14.1   Causes of syncope

Vascular
- Vasovagal ('simple') faint
- Abnormal vagal tone
- Reflex anoxic seizure
- Orthostatic hypotension
- Carotid sinus hypersensitivity

Cardiac
- Structural
  - Aortic stenosis
  - Hypertrophic cardiomyopathy
  - Pulmonary hypertension
  - Fallot's tetralogy

- Arrhythmia
  - Complete heart block
  - Sinus node dysfunction
  - Ventricular tachycardia
  - Long QT syndrome
  - Supraventricular tachycardia

Miscellaneous
- Hyperventilation
- Breath holding
- Obstructive apnoea

Sudden death   Sudden death in children older than 1 year of age is rare and heart disease accounts for some cases. However, asthma, epilepsy and infection are commoner causes. Hypertrophic cardiomyopathy, aortic stenosis and coronary artery abnormalities are most frequently implicated. If cardiac disease is identified or if the absence of another diagnosis points to an arrhythmia, thought should be given to family screening.

Sudden death late after cardiac surgery is well recognized. Senning and Mustard procedures for transposition of the great arteries used to be the most frequently encountered group but now that the switch operation has superseded them there are few children in the paediatric age range with this type of anatomy. Sudden death in patients after tetralogy of Fallot repair is recognized and is dealt with later in this chapter.

Sinus node dysfunction   The sinus node lies at the junction of the superior vena cava and the right atrium. Sinus node dysfunction (SND) may be autonomic, drug-induced or due to structural abnormalities. The term 'sick sinus syndrome' is sometimes used synonymously.

The surface electrocardiogram cannot detect the depolarization of the sinus node, but its function is inferred from the atrial depolarization (P

Table 14.2 Causes of sinus node dysfunction

Group	Example
Idiopathic/congenital	
Familial	
Congenital heart disease	Atrial septal defects
	Atrioventricular septal defects
Cardiomyopathies	
Inflammatory	Rheumatic fever
Ischaemic	Kawasaki's disease
Drugs	Antiarrhythmic agents
	Vagotonic agents
Endocrine/metabolic	Hypoxia
	Hypothyroidism
Increased vagal tone	Idiopathic (reflex anoxic seizure)
	Nasopharyngeal stimulation
	Sleep
	Breath holding
	Increased intracranial pressure
	Drugs (parasympathomimetics)
Surgical	Atrial operations

wave). Arrhythmias due to SND can be slow, fast or irregular. Bradyarrhythmias are due to sinus bradycardia, pause or arrest or to sinoatrial exit block where the conduction from the sinus node to the atria is prolonged. Sinus arrhythmia may be exaggerated in SND. Tachyarrhythmias are caused by sinus node and atrial muscle re-entry.

Bradycardia is hard to define, but on the basis of Holter monitoring studies it is reasonable to suggest that a heart rate below 60 in a child under 6 years, below 45 in a 7–11-year-old and below 40 in someone over 12 is abnormal at any time, including sleep, and warrants careful evaluation. Severe sinus arrhythmia is diagnosed when the R–R interval varies by more than 100%. It must be remembered that just because the heart rate is outside the norm it does not necessarily mean that treatment is indicated.

AETIOLOGY

There are many causes of SND; these are listed with examples in Table 14.2. A significant number are unexplained and there are rare reports of familial occurrence.

The most common cause of sinus node dysfunction in the paediatric population remains iatrogenic after cardiac surgery. Cardiac bypass and ischaemic arrest may be sufficient to damage the sinus node, but it is most commonly seen after surgical procedures on the atria.

PRESENTATION

Most people with sinus node dysfunction remain asymptomatic. The most common symptoms are either fatigue and exercise intolerance or dizziness and syncope. The manifestations of these symptoms will obviously depend on the age of the child. Ideally the symptomatic episodes should be captured on Holter monitoring (Figures 14.2, 14.3).

TREATMENT

As the most common cause remains iatrogenic after surgery, prevention is one of the most important ways of reducing its incidence. Improved surgical technique and understanding of the anatomy and blood supply of the sinus node have led to a decrease in the incidence.

In the short term atropine or isoprenaline are usually effective whatever the cause. The success of long-term drug treatment is variable and side effects from the drugs are usually unacceptable.

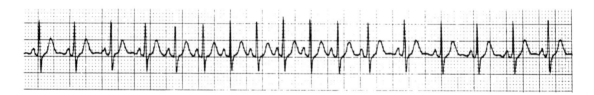

Figure 14.2   ECG showing sinus arrhythmia as heart rate varies with respiration in a patient with raised intracranial pressure. (All ECGs in this section have been recorded with a paper speed of 25 mm/s and 1 mV = 10 mm.)

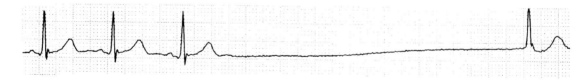

Figure 14.3   ECG showing a sinus pause with a ventricular escape beat after 4 s.

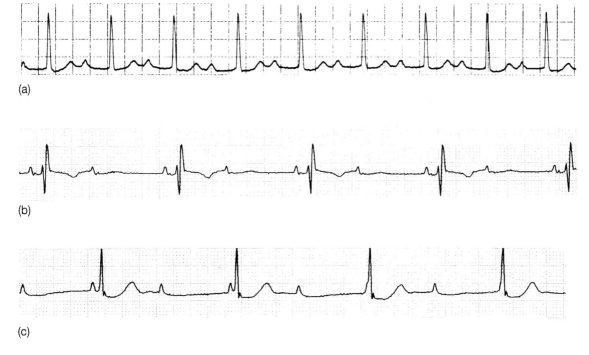

(a)

(b)

(c)

Figure 14.4   ECGs demonstrating the different kinds of heart block. (a) First-degree heart block with a prolonged P–R interval of 320 ms. (b) Second-degree heart block with 2:1 conduction. (c) Complete heart block with an atrial rate of 80 beats/min and a ventricular escape rhythm of 39 beats/min.

Implantation of a permanent pacemaker is indicated if long-term treatment for SND is required. The indications for treatment, however, are not so clear-cut. If the child is symptomatic with syncope or near syncope during documented episodes of SND the decision is straightforward. However, recommendations for treatment in children who have either asymptomatic SND or SND with symptoms compatible with dysrhythmia but no documented evidence of a causal relationship are more difficult to make. Most recommendations are arbitrary. There is no evidence to suggest that an asymptomatic sinus bradycardia above 30 beats/min in children over 6 years is associated with sudden death. It therefore seems reasonable not to insert pacemakers into these patients. However, indications in younger children or those with bradycardias below 30 beats/min remain controversial. Children with SND who require antiarrhythmic drugs for tachyarrhythmias require pacing.

FIRST-DEGREE HEART BLOCK   **Atrioventricular block**

This (Figure 14.4(a)) is defined as an abnormally long P–R interval for the patient's age.

The P–R interval is shorter than 160 ms in infancy, rising to a maximum of 180 ms in adolescents. Its significance lies in its association with a number of disease states, including rheumatic fever, hypothermia, electrolyte disturbances, congenital heart disease and some muscular dystrophies. While it is generally regarded as being benign it can be progressive and there are familial cases associated with sudden death.

SECOND-DEGREE HEART BLOCK

This (Figure 14.4(b)) is divided into to Mobitz type 1 and 2. Mobitz type 1 block displays the Wenckebach phenomenon, in which the P–R interval progressively increases until there is a non-conducted P wave. This is seen in normal individuals while asleep. It is usually asymptomatic and stable and requires no treatment. Mobitz type 2 block consists of intermittent non-conduction of P waves without a variation in the P–R interval of those that are conducted. Usually the block follows a regular pattern in the form of 2:1 or 3:1 block. In the paediatric population it is most commonly seen after surgery. Its importance lies in the fact that it can be progressive and the patient may develop complete heart block.

COMPLETE HEART BLOCK

Complete heart block occurs when the atrial impulse cannot propagate to the ventricles (Figure 14.4(c)). In the paediatric population it is usually either congenital or occurs after surgery (Table 14.3).

The incidence of congenital block is reported at 1/22 000 live births. It is found in association with structural heart lesions, especially congenitally corrected transposition. It may be associated with anti-Ro antibodies in the mother but the exact mechanism by which these

Table 14.3   Causes of complete heart block

Congenital
- Idiopathic
- Maternal connective tissue disease (mother may be asymptomatic)
- Strucural heart disease (often complex)
- Long QT syndrome (may be familial)

Acquired
- Hypertrophic cardiomyopathy
- Myotonic dystrophy
- Infective (myocarditis, rheumatic fever, diphtheria, Lyme disease)
- Following cardiac surgery

---

antibodies affect the His bundle is not known. While some studies have shown 75% of all neonates with complete heart block and structurally normal hearts have been exposed to anti-Ro antibodies, not all positive mothers have babies with complete heart block.

There is a great variation in symptoms in children with complete heart block, from exercise intolerance, syncope, congestive heart failure and even sudden death to a total lack of symptoms. An ECG is all that is required to make the diagnosis. The diagnosis can be made antenatally with fetal echocardiography.

Drug treatment of the bradycardia is disappointing, although isoprenaline and atropine may be used in an emergency situation to speed up the ventricular escape rhythm. Heart failure should be treated with diuretics and inotropes as appropriate. Pacing is the mainstay of treatment and is performed on all symptomatic individuals and those with associated congenital structural lesions. There are large and consistent studies showing that asymptomatic neonates with a ventricular escape rhythm faster than 55 beats/min are at low risk of sudden death. Most units therefore recommend pacemaker insertion in those whose heart rate is slower than 55 beats/min. Epicardial pacemaker leads are used predominantly in neonates and infants, but in an emergency temporary transoesophageal or transvenous pacing may be used.

In the older child pacemaker insertion is recommended in those with a decreased exercise tolerance, with awake heart rates of less than 45 beats/min and with syncope or near syncope.

Improvements in surgical technique have reduced the incidence of postoperative complete heart block. Temporary pacing wires are inserted at the time of surgery. If the patient is still in complete heart block 10–14 days postoperatively most centres would recommend insertion of a permanent pacemaker system.

Bundle branch block

Bundle branch block represents abnormal depolarization through the bundle of His. It causes abnormally wide QRS complexes due to delayed depolarization of the intraventricular conduction tissue. A preexcitation ECG (see Figure 14.10) can be confused with bundle branch block. Right bundle branch (see Figure 14.13) block is most commonly due to a surgical ventriculotomy. Left bundle branch block is rarer and can be caused by cardiomyopathy and severe left ventricular outflow obstruction. Rarely, no pathological cause for the left bundle branch block is found; in these circumstances it can be intermittent.

Atrial arrhythmias

Premature atrial contractions (Figure 14.5) have been reported in up to 21% of healthy children. If they occur in isolation no further investigations or treatment are necessary.

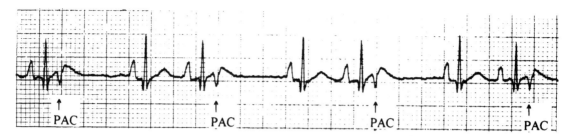

Figure 14.5   Rhythm strip demonstrating non-conducted premature atrial contractions (PAC).

Chaotic atrial rhythms are occasionally seen in infants. They are characterized by multiple (at least three) morphologies of P waves, and are often asymptomatic.

ATRIAL FLUTTER

Atrial flutter appears on the ECG as 'saw-tooth' P waves (Figure 14.6).

It is probably due to a re-entry pathway within the atria. It may either be congenital, and can be diagnosed in the fetus, or secondary to surgery, particularly atrial surgery. Only rarely does it occur as an isolated finding later in childhood.

In the fetus 1:1 conduction may occur, resulting in tachycardias of over 300 beats/min, causing hydrops. Treatment is with digoxin for the mother, and early delivery may be considered. Postnatally direct current synchronized cardioversion restores sinus rhythm although relapses may occur. Further treatment with digoxin may be necessary but the condition is usually self-limiting.

In the older child synchronized cardioversion also works, but relapses are common. Digoxin alone may not be sufficient and further anti-arrhythmic agents may need to be added. As an alternative to cardio-version, overdrive pacing of the flutter frequently works. There are now pacemakers that can overdrive these arrhythmias automatically but there is little experience of their use in the paediatric population.

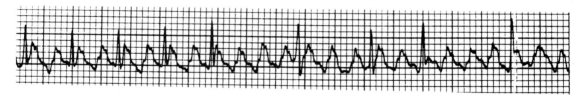

Figure 14.6   ECG demonstrating atrial flutter with the characteristic 'saw tooth' undulating P waves.

Transcatheter ablation is used in the treatment of adults with atrial flutter but not yet in children.

ATRIAL FIBRILLATION

This is very rare in children. Hyperthyroidism should be sought but is very rarely found. Structural and heart muscle disease should be excluded. Isolated sustained or paroxysmal atrial fibrillation can be familial. Cardioversion can restore sinus rhythm but relapse rates are high, depending on aetiology. Pharmacological prophylaxis may involve a variety of drugs. Anticoagulation needs to be considered and is always appropriate for some weeks prior to cardioversion.

Supraventricular tachycardias

Supraventricular tachycardia (SVT) is the commonest symptomatic arrhythmia in children, affecting between 1/250 and 1/1000 children. It is usually defined as a tachycardia originating proximal to the bifurcation of the bundle of His. Typically, the tachycardia is narrow complex and is often faster than 230 beats/min (Figure 14.7); however there are exceptions to this. If the ventricles are not stimulated in the usual manner through the AV node and His bundle, conduction is said to be aberrant and the resulting QRS complex may be broad.

The mechanisms for generation of the tachycardia vary but can be subdivided into three groups illustrated and described in Figure 14.8.

ATRIAL ECTOPIC FOCUS

Ectopic focus

This accounts for a significant number of patients with SVT, particularly in younger age groups. Treatment with drugs rarely restores sinus rhythm although the tachycardia can be slowed down with digoxin and beta-blockers. If the ectopic focus can be localized during an electrophysiology study it can be ablated, although on occasions this just unmasks multiple ectopic foci.

Figure 14.7   Onset of a supraventricular tachycardia recorded on a 24 h tape. Note the atrial premature contraction (APC), which initiates the re-entry circuit (see text for detailed explanation). The QRS complexes are of narrow morphology and the P waves can be seen buried in the T waves.

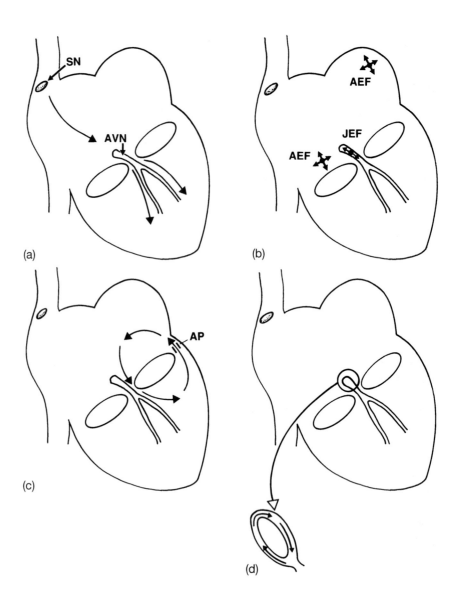

Figure 14.8   Representation of the mechanisms of supraventricular tachycardias (see text for detailed explanation). **(a)** Sinus rhythm with the electrical impulse travelling down from the sinus node (SN) to the atrioventricular node (AVN) and into the ventricles down the His bundle. **(b)** Supraventricular tachycardias can be caused by ectopic foci anywhere in the atria (atrial ectopic focus – AEF) or from a junctional ectopic focus (JEF). **(c)** The commonest mechanism of SVT in children is an AV re-entry circuit through an accessory pathway (AP). **(d)** AV node re-entry tachycardias are cause by a circuit involving the AV node and para-AV nodal fibres.

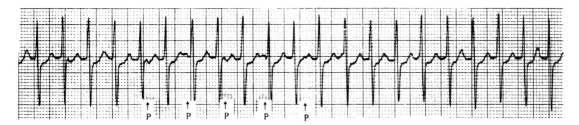

Figure 14.9   ECG showing a junctional ectopic SVT (**His bundle tachycardia**) in which P waves can be seen dissociated from and slower than QRS complexes.

JUNCTIONAL ECTOPIC FOCUS

This condition is rare and unique to the paediatric population. It is most commonly seen in the postoperative period. The focus lies in the AV node/His bundle area, hence the alternative term – 'His bundle tachycardia' (Figure 14.9).

The ECG shows a narrow QRS complex with AV dissociation with sinus P waves (slower than the ventricular rate) 'marching' through the tracing. Occasionally there may be 1:1 ventriculoatrial conduction, with P waves just visible buried in the T wave. It is very resistant to treatment and can be fatal in a compromised postoperative patient.

Overdrive pacing works on some occasions. Junctional ectopic focus does not usually respond to drug treatment, although limited success has been reported with sotalol, amiodarone, flecainide, phenytoin and propafenone. Successful and permanent treatment with surgical or transcatheter radiofrequency ablation has also been reported. Postoperatively this SVT is usually transient and the most successful management has been achieved by reducing chronotropic drugs and cooling the patient down to 34–36°C to lower the heart rate and protect the organs from the poor cardiac output until sinus rhythm returns spontaneously. This can be combined with atrial pacing to restore AV synchrony and increase cardiac output.

Re-entry *via* an accessory pathway

These SVTs are propagated by a re-entry circuit involving a bypass tract connecting the atria and ventricles.

WOLFF–PARKINSON–WHITE SYNDROME

Wolff–Parkinson–White syndrome (WPW; Figure 14.10) is characterized by a short P–R interval due to rapid anterograde (from atria to

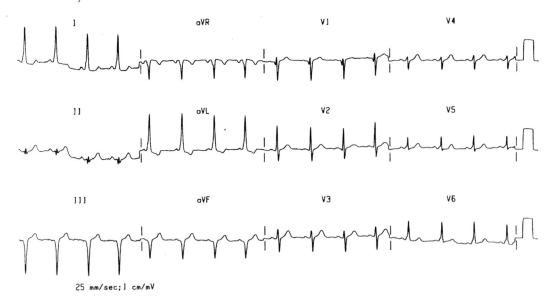

Figure 14.10   Resting ECG showing the characteristic features of Wolff–Parkinson–White syndrome with a short P–R interval and slurred initial QRS delta wave.

ventricle) conduction and a broad QRS complex caused by premature activation of the ventricle through the accessory pathway followed by normal depolarization of the ventricle through the AV node and bundle of His.

The majority of cases exist in otherwise structurally normal hearts, although there is an association with Ebstein's anomaly of the tricuspid valve. Sporadic familial cases have been reported and there is a slightly increased incidence in males. Overall incidence in healthy subjects is up to 2/1000.

Unidirectional retrograde accessory pathway (sometimes called concealed WPW syndrome) occurs when the accessory pathway can only conduct retrogradely. The resting ECG is therefore normal.

Intermittent Wolff–Parkinson–White syndrome is due to an accessory pathway that only conducts anterogradely in certain clinical conditions or in the catheter laboratory. There is a normal resting ECG.

LOWN–GANONG–LEVINE SYNDROME

This is thought to have an accessory pathway running from the atria directly into the bundle of His, bypassing the AV node, hence the characteristic short P–R interval with a normal QRS complex.

PERMANENT JUNCTIONAL RECIPROCATING TACHYCARDIA

This involves a posteroseptal accessory pathway and is associated with narrow QRS complexes during the tachycardia. It is the most common form of incessant SVT in children and may present with features similar to dilated cardiomyopathy.

MAHAIM SVT

This condition is uncommon. It involves a right accessory AV node inserting into right bundle fibres. This results in broad QRS complexes with left bundle branch block morphology both during sinus rhythm (with a normal P–R interval) and during SVT.

MECHANISM OF ARRHYTHMIA

The refractory period of the AV node is usually shorter than that of the accessory pathway and therefore allows anterograde conduction sooner. Therefore, if an atrial ectopic occurs soon after a sinus atrial depolarization (Figure 14.7) it travels through the AV node while the accessory pathway remains refractory and stimulates the ventricle. By the time the ventricular depolarization has reached the accessory pathway it is ready to conduct again and will do so retrogradely. Thus a re-entry circuit is set up as follows: anterograde through the AV node, bundle of His, ventricular myocardium, retrograde through accessory pathway, atrium and back to the AV node (orthodromic reciprocating tachycardia). The ventricular myocardium is being stimulated by the normal means through the bundle of His and so the QRS complexes are narrow. Rarely, the re-entry circuit is the reverse: i.e. anterograde through the accessory pathway to the ventricular myocardium, retrograde through the bundle of His and AV node, back to the atrium and the accessory pathway again (antidromic reciprocating tachycardia). This gives a broad complex QRS SVT with inverted P waves.

If the refractory period of the accessory pathway is short and the patient develops atrial flutter or fibrillation (uncommon in children) this can result in rapid conduction of impulses to the ventricle. This can be fatal. Drugs that decrease the refractory period of the accessory pathway are therefore potentially dangerous. For this reason digoxin is contraindicated in older children with AV accessory pathways unless the refractory period is known to be long. Digoxin appears to be safe in infants although the reason for this is not entirely clear.

TREATMENT

Some episodes of SVT are well tolerated and can be allowed to revert spontaneously. If the SVT needs to be terminated acutely (Figure 14.11), this can be done with vagal manoeuvres in a large proportion of children. Facial immersion in ice cold water is very effective in infants (Figure 14.12).

Older children can often terminate the SVT by performing a Valsalva manoeuvre or by placing an ice pack (or a packet of frozen peas) over the face or eating ice-cream. Carotid sinus massage has a disappointingly low success rate. Ocular pressure is generally discouraged because of the theoretical possibility of retinal detachment.

Adenosine by rapid IV injection is a very effective way of terminating re-entry tachycardias. The initial dose is 0.05 mg/kg, increasing by 0.05 mg/kg per dose until the SVT is terminated or a maximum dose of 0.25 mg/kg is reached. Adenosine can cause sinus bradycardia or AV block if given in high doses. Sinus arrest may occur if the child already has sinus node dysfunction. Full resuscitation equipment must therefore

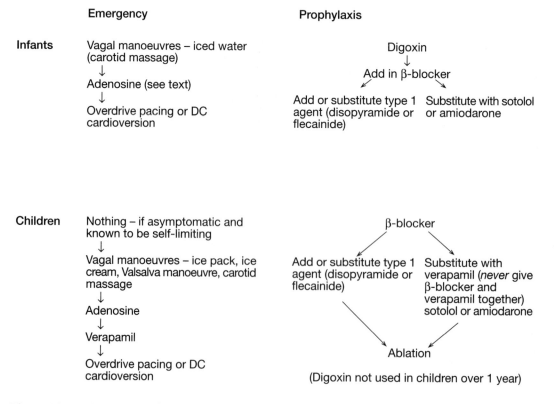

Figure 14.11   Treatment of SVT.

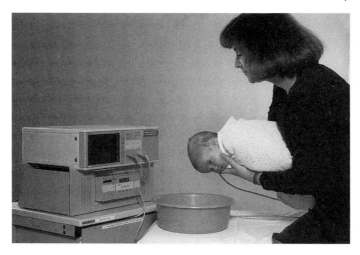

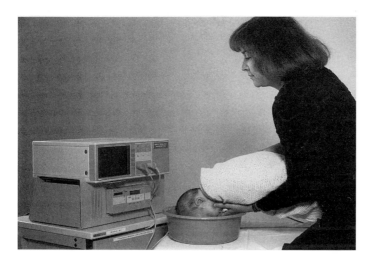

Figure 14.12   Simulated facial immersion in cold water for treatment of SVT in young infants. Notice ECG monitor, which is interfaced to a running paper printer. (Reproduced from Archer, N. (1995) Management of supraventricular tachycardia. *Current Paediatrics*, **5**, 59–63, with permission from the publishers, Churchill Livingstone).

be available when administering adenosine. It may also cause dyspnoea, coughing or bronchoconstriction in asthmatics, and flushing, headache and agitation. Concurrent dipyridamole therapy enhances and extends adenosine's effect and there is an important risk of toxicity.

In exceptional circumstances overdrive pacing, either *via* a trans-oesophageal electrode or with an intracardiac lead may be considered.

Synchronized cardioversion (under heavy sedation or general anaesthesia) is also frequently successful and should be used in a severely compromised patient in whom adenosine has failed.

In a few cases there is an obvious precipitant (e.g. caffeine) and this can be avoided. Long-term prophylaxis should be started if there is any cardiac compromise associated with episodes or if the frequency of them is becoming debilitating to the child. A number of children with WPW syndrome, especially if they present in infancy, stop having SVTs either with or without resolution of pre-excitation, if present. Any treatment modality, particularly if started in infancy, must be reassessed by weaning it off at intervals as it may no longer be required.

In infants digoxin remains the treatment of choice. It slows conduction across the normal AV node but does not target the abnormal accessory pathway. In older children it is contraindicated (see above). Beta-blockers are the mainstay of prophylactic drug treatment of SVT after infancy.

If single therapy does not control the SVT another agent can be either substituted or added (Figure 14.11).

Transcatheter radiofrequency ablation of the accessory pathway is now a well established procedure in adult practice. It is not without its risks, but may be considered in those whose SVT continues past infancy and is not easily controlled with well tolerated drugs.

Re-entry without a bypass tract

AV NODE RE-ENTRY TACHYCARDIA

AV node re-entry tachycardia is the second most common cause of SVT in the paediatric population (and the commonest in adults). It is rare in young children and most frequently presents at the time of puberty. The circuit for the development of the tachycardia consists of an anterograde limb through the AV node with the retrograde limb through para-AV nodal fibres which, despite their name, can lie at some distance from the AV node. The ECG during the tachycardia shows narrow QRS complexes and a P wave can often be seen immediately after the QRS complexes.

This SVT is particularly susceptible to vagal manoeuvres and so it can usually be controlled adequately by the patient performing a Valsalva manoeuvre. If the attacks are infrequent this may be sufficient treatment. In the acute phase almost 100% of attacks can be terminated with adenosine. Prophylaxis is usually achieved with digoxin. Verapamil has been used frequently in adults but is usually avoided in infants as it can be fatal if given in the presence of poor ventricular function. Recently, interest has revolved around ablating the extra AV nodal structure. In experienced hands this has a high success rate, a low complication rate and is curative, and obviates the need for lifelong drug therapy.

SINUS NODE RE-ENTRY TACHYCARDIA AND ATRIAL MUSCLE RE-ENTRY TACHYCARDIA

These are also rare. They can be difficult to differentiate from an atrial ectopic focus. The arrhythmia may be very persistent and lead to cardiac decompensation. The ECG shows a normal QRS complex but the P wave axis may be abnormal. Adenosine, if used, will produce AV block and reveal the atrial tachycardia. The ventricular rate may be controlled with digoxin but control of the atrial rate can be difficult. Success has been achieved with flecainide, amiodarone and sotalol. Again transcatheter ablation may offer a cure for this arrhythmia.

OTHERS

Atrial flutter and atrial fibrillation have already been discussed (pp. 148–9).

Ventricular arrhythmias

Ventricular arrhythmias originate distal to the bifurcation of the bundle of His and have many causes (Table 14.4). They can be broadly divided into three categories: premature ventricular contractions, ventricular tachycardia and ventricular fibrillation.

Table 14.4 Acute and chronic causes of ventricular arrhythmias

Group	Example
Idiopathic	
Metabolic	Hypoxia
	Acidosis
	Electrolyte imbalances
Congenital	Long QT syndrome
	Congenital heart disease
Acquired	Cardiomyopathies
	Cardiac tumours
	Ischaemic (e.g. Kawasaki disease)
Iatrogenic	Postoperative
Infective	Myocarditis
	Rheumatic fever

PREMATURE VENTRICULAR CONTRACTIONS

Premature ventricular contractions (PVC) are also known as **ventricular ectopics, extrasystoles** or **premature beats**. By definition they occur earlier than expected, usually with abnormal QRS morphology and duration, and have no preceding P wave (Figure 14.13). They should be differentiated from a premature atrial contraction with aberrant conduction, which would be preceded by a premature P wave.

PVCs can be either **uniform** if they all have the same morphology or **multiform** if they exhibit different morphologies. Care should be taken to differentiate multiform PVCs from a fusion beat where the ventricle is activated simultaneously from the atria *via* the bundle of His and from the PVC. Fusion beats will therefore be preceded by a P wave and show intermediate morphology between a PVC and a sinus QRS complex. PVCs may occur regularly every second or third complex producing **bigeminy** or **trigeminy** respectively. **Couplets** are two PVCs without an intervening normal QRS complex.

Premature ventricular contractions are often normal and require no further action if:

- the ECG is otherwise normal;
- the child is asymptomatic;
- cardiovascular examination is normal;
- they disappear with modest exertion;
- there is no family history suggestive of serious arrhythmias.

They can, however, be a marker for cardiac pathology (see under ventricular tachycardia). It is therefore reasonable to perform an echocardiogram on those children who do not fulfil the above criteria. In addition, 24-hour Holter monitoring and exercise testing are indicated, looking for more serious arrhythmias that may even be precipitated by exercise. While drug treatment may reduce the frequency of the PVCs it must be remembered that treatment with antiarrhythmics is not without

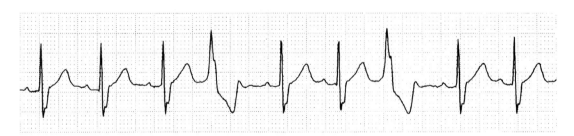

Figure 14.13   ECG from a postoperative patient showing two premature ventricular contractions. Note that the QRS morphology is different from the sinus beats and is not preceded by a P wave. The sinus beats show right bundle branch block following a right ventriculotomy.

its hazards. Therefore, if these investigations are normal and the child is asymptomatic, treatment is not indicated even if the PVCs are frequent.

VENTRICULAR TACHYCARDIA

Ventricular tachycardia is defined as three or more consecutive beats originating in the ventricle distal to the bifurcation of the bundle of His. The QRS morphology is different from that in sinus rhythm and normally shows ventriculoatrial dissociation (Figure 14.14). Its rate is usually greater than 120 beats/min.

Clinically the child may be asymptomatic or present with syncope or near syncope. The diagnosis is usually obvious on an ECG obtained while symptomatic. It must, however, be differentiated from an SVT with aberrant conduction, which is uncommon unless bundle branch block exists when in sinus rhythm. Adenosine can be used to differentiate these broad complex tachycardias, as AV block caused by its administration will usually restore to sinus rhythm or slow down SVT but have no effect on ventricular tachycardias.

Ventricular tachycardia with a normal heart

This may occur from infancy onwards, but a detailed search for an underlying cause must always be made (Table 14.4). Thus, detailed echocardiography is always indicated and cardiac catheterization may be performed to look for subtle features of arrhythmogenic right ventricular dysplasia. If the patient is asymptomatic and no cause is found drug treatment is not necessarily indicated. **Incessant idiopathic ventricular tachycardia** is defined as VT present for at least 10% of the time. It is usually seen in infants and is often almost continuous. Incessant idiopathic VT is characteristically associated with a ventricular hamartoma. It may respond to flecainide or amiodarone and eventually resolves spontaneously. Surgery, once commonly used, is occasionally needed.

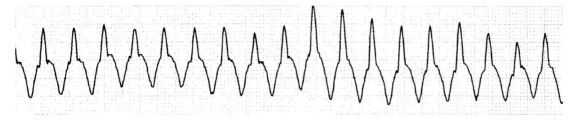

Figure 14.14 Recording from a Holter monitor showing ventricular tachycardia at a rate of approximately 170 beats/min.

Congenital heart disease

Unoperated congenital heart disease is associated with an increased incidence of ventricular arrhythmias. **Mitral valve prolapse** is relatively common in the general population and is associated with an increased incidence of arrhythmias. Treatment is not recommended in the absence of symptoms from the arrhythmias. **Ebstein's anomaly** is associated not only with WPW syndrome but also with ventricular arrhythmias. Sudden death in this group appears to be relatively common and so treatment for arrhythmias is indicated even in the absence of symptoms. **Tetralogy of Fallot** may be associated with ventricular arrhythmias before correction, although surgery is now usually early enough to avoid this phase of the natural history (see postoperative arrhythmias, below).

Rhabdomyomas and other ventricular tumours in children are rare, but have been associated with ventricular arrhythmias and should be treated. It should be remembered that cardiac rhabdomyomas can be the presenting feature of tuberous sclerosis.

Cardiomyopathy

Cardiomyopathies of all sorts are associated with ventricular arrhythmias. They are covered in detail in Chapter 11.

Surgery for congenital heart disease

Postoperative congenital heart disease is associated with a variety of arrhythmias, including ventricular tachycardias. Arrhythmias following repair of tetralogy of Fallot have been extensively looked at because it is a common congenital heart defect with a good surgical prognosis. Unfortunately, a number of sudden deaths have been reported in prolonged follow-up studies. It is important to try and identify high-risk groups. A history of symptoms is unreliable as the first episode may be terminal. Holter studies are usually undertaken at follow-up.

There is some controversy about treatment of asymptomatic tachycardias. Symptomatic individuals should always be treated. Recent studies suggest that a QRS interval of greater than 180 ms may be a marker for ventricular tachycardias and may warrant more frequent Holter tapes. Surgery to improve major residual or recurrent haemodynamic abnormalities is indicated.

Poisoning

Poisoning with digoxin and tricyclic antidepressants are specifically associated with ventricular tachycardias. Digoxin poisoning should be treated with the digoxin-specific antibody. If VT occurs, lignocaine or

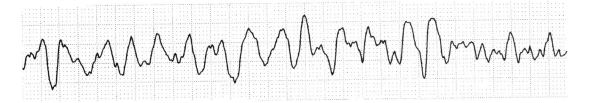

Figure 14.15 **Holter recording** showing ventricular fibrillation.

cardioversion is required. Tricyclic poisoning should be managed with appropriate intensive care support. If the VT causes significant haemodynamic compromise, a short acting beta-blocker such as esmolol is indicated. Lignocaine should be avoided as it may aggravate the arrhythmia. Cardiac massage may be required for many hours, as eventual recovery can still occur.

VENTRICULAR FIBRILLATION

Ventricular fibrillation in paediatrics is rare. It is characterized by uncoordinated ventricular depolarizations with no cardiac output and is not difficult to diagnose providing detached ECG leads are recognized. The ECG shows rapid, low amplitude, irregular depolarizations with no identifiable QRS complexes (Figure 14.15). Treatment is with defibrillation. If this is not successful full cardiopulmonary resuscitation is started (Figure 14.16).

Long QT syndromes are rare congenital disorders associated with serious ventricular arrhythmias. They are characterized by syncope due to ventricular tachycardias in association with a long QT interval. *Torsades de pointes* (Figure 14.17) is the characteristic ventricular tachyarrhythmia, which is almost pathognomonic of the long QT syndromes. The first symptomatic episode is usually in childhood.

Long QT syndromes

Some 25–30% of cases of long QT syndrome are sporadic with no family history. The remaining patients inherit the disorder either as an autosomal dominant condition (Romano–Ward syndrome) or as the rarer autosomal recessive disorder with congenital deafness (Jervell Lange–Neilsen syndrome).

The clinical history is almost diagnostic, with repeated episodes of syncope associated with emotional stress, frequently due to a sudden fright or physical stress.

A long QT interval is not always obvious on the ECG (Figure 14.18) and should be specifically looked for.

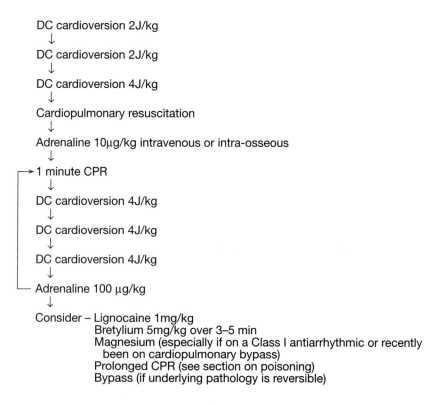

DC cardioversion 2J/kg
↓
DC cardioversion 2J/kg
↓
DC cardioversion 4J/kg
↓
Cardiopulmonary resuscitation
↓
Adrenaline 10µg/kg intravenous or intra-osseous
↓
1 minute CPR
↓
DC cardioversion 4J/kg
↓
DC cardioversion 4J/kg
↓
DC cardioversion 4J/kg
↓
Adrenaline 100 µg/kg
↓
Consider – Lignocaine 1mg/kg
           Bretylium 5mg/kg over 3–5 min
           Magnesium (especially if on a Class I antiarrhythmic or recently
              been on cardiopulmonary bypass)
           Prolonged CPR (see section on poisoning)
           Bypass (if underlying pathology is reversible)

Figure 14.16   Treatment of ventricular fibrillation/pulseless ventricular tachycardia in accordance with Resuscitation Council UK guidelines 1997.

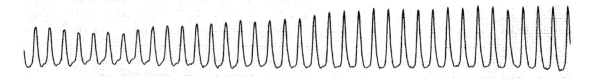

Figure 14.17   Rhythm strip showing *torsades de pointes* (polymorphic ventricular tachycardia). Note the sinusoidal pattern of the QRS complexes as they gradually shift from negative to positive.

A corrected QT interval (QT$_c$) can be calculated.

$$QT_c = \frac{measured QT}{\sqrt{RR}}$$

The QT interval (in seconds) is measured from the start of the Q wave to the end of the T wave. The RR interval measured is the one

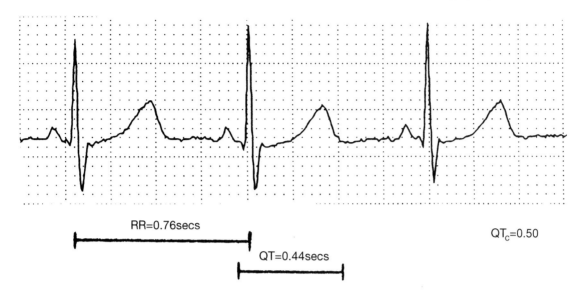

RR=0.76secs

QT=0.44secs

QT$_c$=0.50

Figure 14.18   Rhythm strip from a Holter recording. A prolonged QT$_c$ may not always be obvious on the ECG and must be specifically measured. This rhythm strip was taken from a 6-year-old child who presented after a near-drowning.

immediately preceding the QRS complex whose QT interval has been measured. QT$_c$ longer than 0.44 is considered abnormal. The ECG may also show sinus bradycardia and an alternating T wave axis. However, long QT$_c$ intervals have been reported in normal infants, and in older children when asleep or those with marked sinus arrhythmia. It should also be borne in mind that it is possible to have episodes of *torsades de pointes* despite having a QT$_c$ less than 0.44.

A great deal of research is at present being undertaken to look at the genetic and molecular mechanisms of the long QT syndromes. It is hypothesized that abnormalities of ion flux in cardiac tissues are responsible. A number of the genes responsible have been identified and as their function is elucidated it may be possible to direct treatment at specific molecular abnormalities. As most long QT syndromes appear to be catecholamine-driven, treatment at present is aimed at reducing sympathetic innervation of the heart. Pharmacologically this is achieved with beta-blockers, usually propranolol, and is effective in 75–80% of patients. Patients in whom beta-blockade is ineffective may benefit from a left cardiac sympathetic denervation.

In those patients who become symptomatically bradycardic on beta-blockers or in whom long pauses are seen on Holter monitoring, a pacemaker may need to be inserted to relieve symptoms. Pacemakers may also play a therapeutic role in protecting against the development of *torsades de pointes*.

Recently, implantable cardioverter defibrillators (ICD) have become small enough to implant into children. This would be a last resort and great care must be taken to assess patients before this is contemplated. It is extremely unpleasant to be cardioverted while still awake. This and the fear of the underlying diagnosis can result in severe psychological stress.

ACQUIRED LONG QT SYNDROMES

There are several conditions that can prolong the QT interval in a healthy individual and if these conditions occur in someone with a long QT syndrome they are more likely to develop arrhythmias.

Electrolyte imbalances, especially hypocalcaemia and hypomagnesaemia, prolong the QT interval. Drug-induced prolongation of the QT interval is well recognized, and patients with prolonged QT syndrome should be advised to avoid these drugs. They include antiarrhythmics (quinidine, procainamide, disopyramide, amiodarone and sotalol), most antipsychotics, antihistamines (terfenadine and astemizole – others appear to be safe), some antimalarials, cisapride and erythromycin. Central nervous system trauma, especially subarachnoid haemorrhage, prolongs the QT interval. Primary myocardial dysfunction due to myocarditis or ischaemia can also prolong the QT interval and is associated with ventricular arrhythmias.

Table 14.5 Information on antiarrhythmic drugs mentioned in text (all drug doses are given as total daily dose unless otherwise stated)

Drug	Dose	Notes
Adenosine	Rapid IV bolus – initially 0.05 mg/kg increasing by 0.05 mg/kg to a maximum of 0.25 mg/kg if no effect achieved	Used to terminate SVTs that involve the atrioventricular node as part of the re-entry circuit. Can also be used diagnostically to differentiate broad complex SVT from a ventricular tachycardia. Can also reveal atrial flutter or primary atrial tachycardias by causing transient AV block.
Amiodarone	Oral maintenance – 150 mg/m^2 Oral loading – 350 mg/m^2 IV infusion – 5 mg/kg over 1 h followed by 10 mg/kg/d	Has a broad antiarrhythmic spectrum. Rarely used as first line treatment. Useful in SVT, atrial and ventricular arrhythmias. Long-term use is complicated by corneal microdeposits, rashes, deranged thyroid function and other less common side-effects. Interacts with many drugs, but particular care should be taken if patients are already on digoxin.
Atropine	IV bolus – 15–20 μg/kg	Used to increase heart rate in sinus node dysfunction or heart block.
Bretylium	IV – 5 mg/kg over 3–5 min	Used for ventricular fibrillation or tachycardia resistant to lignocaine.
Digoxin	Maintenance – 8–10 μg/kg (5–10 μg/kg in preterm) Loading – IV or oral 25–35 μg/kg (20 μg/kg in preterm) give 1/2 dose stat followed by 1/4 dose 8 h and 16 h later	Used to control paroxysmal SVT, atrial flutter and fibrillation. Avoid in atrial flutter or fibrillation with an accessory pathway as may predispose to ventricular tachycardia/fibrillation. For this reason not recommended in children over 1 year.
Disopyramide	Oral – 10–20 mg/kg in three divided dose (two divided doses if using slow release preparation)	Used principally to treat paroxysmal SVT but also effective in atrial flutter/fibrillation and ventricular arrhythmias.
Esmolol	IV – 600 μg/kg over 1 min	Very short acting β-blocker useful in the emergency treatment of atrial tachyarrhythmias or ventricular tachycardia due to tricyclic poisoning.
Flecainide	Oral – 3–6 mg/kg in two or three divided doses	Used to treat SVT and ventricular arrhythmias as second line treatment.
Isoprenaline	IV infusion – 0.02–0.2 μg/kg/min	Used to increase heart rate in sinus node dysfunction or heart block.
Lignocaine	IV bolus – 1 mg/kg IV maintenance – 20–50 μg/kg/min	Used as emergency treatment of life threatening ventricular arrhythmias.
Phenytoin	IV loading 20 mg/kg over 30 min Oral loading – 15 mg/kg in four divided doses day 1, 7.5 mg/kg in four divided doses day 2 Oral maintenance – approx. 5 mg/kg in two divided doses	Used to control ventricular arrhythmias in patients with structural heart disease or postoperatively. Plasma drug levels should be 12–25 mg/l.

Table 14.5 *cont.*

Drug	Dose	Notes
Propanolol	Oral – 3 mg/kg in three divided doses	Used to treat SVT and ventricular tachycardia (particularly in prolonged QT interval). May also be useful in slowing the heart rate down in atrial flutter and fibrillation. **Never** give with verapamil.
Sotolol	Oral – 2–8 mg/kg in two divided doses.	Similar action and uses to propranolol but also prolongs refractoriness. Therefore more effective in atrial arrhythmias. May be effective against a junctional ectopic focus (His bundle tachycardia).
Verapamil	IV slow bolus – 75–150 µg/kg Oral – 4–10 mg/kg in three divided doses	Should **not** be administered to children already on a β-blocker or infants because of its potentially profound negative inotropic effect. IV verapamil is useful in the acute management of SVT in children. Oral verapamil can be used as a second-line treatment for SVTs or atrial flutter/fibrillation.

Part Five
Specific Lesions

In this section brief notes are given on structural congenital heart lesions. Details are given under a number of headings: introduction, natural history, clinical features, investigations and treatment. The intention is that the facts given in this section do not then need to be repeated each time particular conditions or groups of conditions are referred to elsewhere in the text. It is also hoped that they will provide a valuable rapid source of information. In the natural history section of each condition, infective endocarditis has not been mentioned but all structural heart lesions, with the exception of isolated uncomplicated ostium secundum or sinus venosus type atrial septal defects, do have an increased risk of infective endocarditis compared with the population as a whole and preventative measures are advised (pp. 116–17).

Left-to-right shunts 15

INTRODUCTION (Figure 15.1)

Atrial septal defects (ASD)

- **Patent foramen ovale** (PFO) is not usually considered abnormal, even if it persists throughout life.
- **Ostium secundum ASD** constitutes 5–10% of congenital heart disease and is also a common association with many more complex lesions. Partial anomalous pulmonary venous drainage (PAPVD) may be present.
- **Sinus venosus ASD** constitutes 10% of ASDs; it occurs more commonly in the upper part of the atrial septum adjacent to SVC, but can be close to IVC. There is a strong association with PAPVD.
- **Ostium primum ASD**: see partial AVSD, below.

NATURAL HISTORY

PFO usually closes. The relationship with paradoxical emboli needs clarifying; PFO gives divers an increased risk of 'the bends'.

Secundum ASD. Spontaneous closure up to 2–3 years of age can occur. Symptoms in childhood are rare; supraventricular arrhythmias, paradoxical emboli, right heart failure and pulmonary vascular disease can occur in adult life. Can remain asymptomatic. Life expectancy virtually normal if closure undertaken in childhood.

Sinus venosus ASD. Spontaneous closure does not occur. Natural history otherwise as for secundum ASD.

CLINICAL FEATURES

There is an absence of sinus arrhythmia. S2 is wide and fixed and there is a pulmonary outflow mid-systolic murmur and often mid-diastolic murmur at the lower left sternal edge (due to increased tricuspid flow).

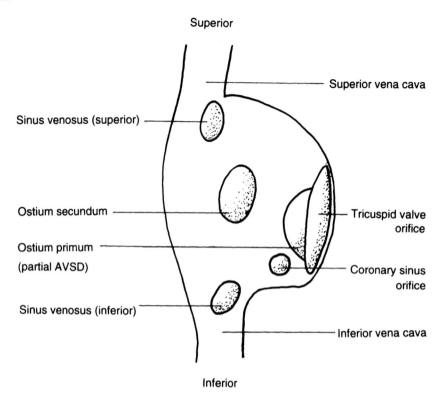

Figure 15.1 Possible sites for atrial septal defects.

INVESTIGATIONS

- **ECG.** rSR in V1. QRS may have right axis deviation.
- **CXR.** Mild cardiomegaly, prominent pulmonary artery, pulmonary plethora.
- **Echocardiogram.** Usually diagnostic, showing location of defect with varying degrees of right heart enlargement. If defect hard to see, transoesophageal echocardiography is helpful.
- **Cardiac catheterization** is rarely necessary.

TREATMENT

If detected in early life closure usually aged 3–4 years or at diagnosis if found in later childhood. Risk/benefit for treatment less clear for those presenting in adult life. Closure is by open heart surgery with very low risk. Long-term risk of arrhythmias is not completely abolished. Transcatheter occlusion is being introduced and is likely to become more widespread.

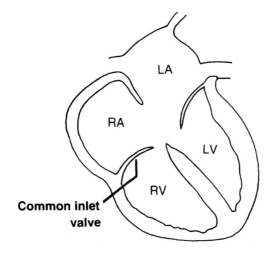

Figure 15.2   Complete atrioventricular septal defect.

Atrioventricular septal defects (AVSD)

INTRODUCTION

- **Partial (ostium primum) AVSD** (Figure 15.1) comprises 1–2% of all congenital heart disease. Atrial shunting occurs; the left atrioventricular (AV) valve is always abnormal and may be regurgitant. Left ventricular to right atrial shunting may occur.
- **Complete AVSD** (Figure 15.2) comprises 2% of congenital heart disease. Strong association with Down's syndrome, which is present in up to 80% of cases (approximately 40% of Down's syndrome people with structural heart disease have complete AVSD). Atrial and ventricular shunting as well as AV regurgitation occur. Occasionally associated with tetralogy of Fallot and coarctation. Often found when there is dextroisomerism.

NATURAL HISTORY

- **Partial AVSD** may develop heart failure and failure to thrive in infancy particularly if AV regurgitation is marked. Pulmonary vascular disease develops in adult life. Some small defects may cause minimal symptoms.
- **Complete AVSD** is very likely to develop heart failure in infancy. Early pulmonary vascular disease is universal and may be irreversible by 1–2 years of age.

CLINICAL FEATURES

- **Partial AVSD.** Signs may be similar to ASD or apical pansystolic murmur of AV regurgitation may dominate.
- **Complete AVSD.** Fixed S2, P2 loud, pansystolic murmur at lower left sternal edge (from VSD) or apex (from AV regurgitation). May have mid-systolic murmur in pulmonary area and mid-diastolic murmur at lower left sternal edge. May have no murmurs.

INVESTIGATIONS

- **ECG**
  - *Partial AVSD*: right atrial enlargement, PR may be prolonged, QRS −30 to −60, rSR V1 with RVH by voltage criteria.
  - *Complete AVSD*: right atrial enlargement, long PR, QRS + 180 to + 270 (north west axis), RVH.
- **CXR.** Both types of AVSD show cardiomegaly, prominent PA and pulmonary plethora.
- **Echocardiogram** is diagnostic in both types and Doppler allows definition of valvar regurgitation.
- **Cardiac catheterization** is only necessary if irreversible pulmonary vascular changes are suspected but not definitely present.

TREATMENT

Aggressive management of heart failure. Surgical closure of partial AVSD necessary in symptomatic infants but can be deferred to 2–4 years of age if well without important pulmonary hypertension. Mortality is less than 5%. Repair of left AV valve usually possible, replacement in childhood only occasionally required.

Complete AVSD should be corrected in early infancy if pulmonary vascular disease is to be avoided. Mortality is less than 10%; left AV valve replacement is rarely needed at primary repair but may be required in later life.

Ventricular septal defect (VSD)

INTRODUCTION

As a single or dominant lesion, VSD represents 32% of structural congenital heart disease, which makes it, with the possible exception of

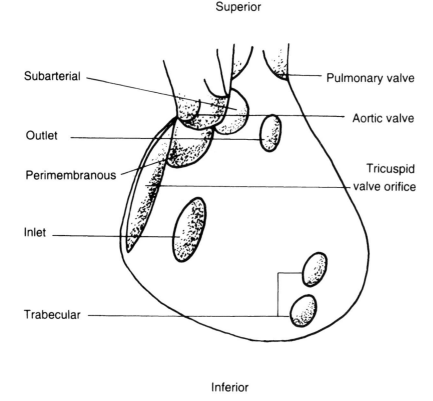

Figure 15.3   Possible sites for ventricular septal defects.

bicuspid aortic valve, the most common structural lesion. VSD is an important part of many more complex anomalies. Defects can be in the inlet, trabecular or outlet septum (Figure 15.3). If adjacent to the central fibrous body of the heart they are termed **perimembranous**.

NATURAL HISTORY

In the region of 65% of VSDs present at birth close spontaneously (some close in fetal life). Others may reduce in size but never close completely. Pathophysiology is that of a left-to-right shunt with increased lung blood flow and/or pressure, which may progress to pulmonary vascular disease if the defect is a large one. Spontaneous closure involves tricuspid valve tissue (so called ventricular septal aneurysm) in perimembranous defects and sometimes the aortic valve cusps producing aortic regurgitation, which can be severe. Progressive muscular subvalvar RV outflow obstruction can develop through infancy, which will reduce lung blood flow and even progress to right-to-left shunting with similar haemodynamics to tetralogy of Fallot.

CLINICAL FEATURES

Small defects are usually asymptomatic, but infants with large defects typically develop heart failure, usually at 2–4 months of age. P2 is loud if pulmonary artery pressure is high. There is typically a 3 or more/6 harsh pansystolic murmur at the lower left sternal edge, often not heard in the immediate newborn period or if pulmonary artery hypertension is marked, or if the hole is large with equalization of pressures. Small defects may be associated with a thrill and a very loud murmur because of the high pressure difference between the ventricles.

If pulmonary blood flow is high (more than twice systemic) a mid-diastolic murmur may be heard at the apex from increased mitral flow. If pulmonary vascular disease develops heart failure and signs of high lung blood flow resolve in the second or third year of life and clinical RVH, loud P2 and quieter or even absent murmur precede the development of late signs – pulmonary regurgitation, cyanosis (Eisenmenger's syndrome), arrhythmias and right heart failure – often by many years.

INVESTIGATIONS

- **ECG**
  - *Small defect*: normal.
  - *Moderate defect*: LVH.
  - *Large defect*: R and LVH.
- **CXR**
  - *Small defect*: normal.
  - *Moderate/large defect*: cardiomegaly, pulmonary plethora.
  - *Pulmonary vascular disease*: large central pulmonary arteries with peripheral pulmonary vessel pruning.
- **Echocardiography** is usually diagnostic.
- **Cardiac catheterization** may be needed to evaluate pulmonary vascular resistance or anatomy if multiple VSDs are suspected.

TREATMENT

Antifailure therapy if indicated. Surgical closure (usually in infancy) is indicated if either failure to thrive in spite of medical therapy or pulmonary artery pressure above half of systemic (usually assessable from ultrasound imaging and Doppler) are present. In older children surgery is indicated if pulmonary blood flow is more than twice systemic, and the defect is getting no smaller or aortic regurgitation or subvalvar pulmonary stenosis develop. Endocarditis is sometimes considered an indication for closure once successfully controlled or treated. There is a very low mortality for VSD closure alone. Pulmonary artery banding is only considered for multiple muscular VSDs in infants or on account of associated lesions such as coarctation or complex anatomy.

INTRODUCTION

Patent ductus arteriosus (PDA)

PDA accounts for 12% of structural congenital heart disease. This figure does not include PDA in association with prematurity and RDS. PDA can accompany virtually any other structural lesion; its presence and the timing of closure affects the clinical picture in many serious lesions (duct-dependent systemic and duct-dependent pulmonary circulations). The haemodynamics of left-to-right shunting exist, with the possibility of pulmonary vascular disease developing if the lesion is not small.

NATURAL HISTORY

For preterm infants see p. 67. Heart failure may develop in infancy. Spontaneous closure after the newborn period in term infants is exceedingly rare. Eisenmenger's complex (p. 134) develops, usually in the second decade or later in large lesions; endocarditis is common in small lesions. Left heart failure can occur in middle age if pulmonary vascular disease has not occurred.

CLINICAL FEATURES

Full pulses, with an active precordium, a continuous murmur under the left clavicle and a diastolic murmur at the apex (from high flow through the mitral valve), are found with or without heart failure in infants. The murmur may be systolic only and colour flow Doppler echocardiography has revealed that some tiny PDAs have no murmur or other signs. If pulmonary vascular disease develops signs of RVH (parasternal heave) will develop and pulses will not be bounding; there may be cyanosed and clubbed toes, but not fingers, due to right-to-left shunting through the defect.

INVESTIGATIONS

- **ECG**
  - *Small defect*: normal.
  - *Moderate defect*: LVH.
  - *Large defect*: R and LVH.
  - *Pulmonary vascular disease*: RVH and strain.
- **CXR**
  - *Small defect*: normal.
  - *Moderate/large defect*: cardiomegaly, pulmonary plethora, large pulmonary artery.
  - *Pulmonary vascular disease*: normal/large heart, peripheral pulmonary vessel pruning, large central pulmonary arteries.
- **Echocardiogram** is usually diagnostic, although difficulties can arise in older children or adults in whom imaging of the arch and duct can be difficult and in whom right-to-left shunting has developed.

TREATMENT

Antifailure therapy should be instituted where appropriate. Closure is recommended for symptomatic infants or if risk of pulmonary vascular disease developing is clear. Asymptomatic infants without right heart hypertension can have closure deferred to the second year of life; in children closure should be performed at diagnosis providing there is not irreversible pulmonary vascular disease, in which circumstance closure is contraindicated. Tiny lesions without physical signs detected co-incidentally on colour flow Doppler probably do not need closing. Closure is by either surgery or transcatheter occlusion. Complete occlusion removes increased risk of infective endocarditis.

Aorto-pulmonary window

INTRODUCTION

This is a rare abnormality in which the ascending aorta has an opening into the main pulmonary artery, allowing left-to-right shunting and transmission of high pressures into the pulmonary artery. PDA may coexist, as may VSD, coarctation or interruption of aorta.

NATURAL HISTORY

Heart failure in infancy and the development of pulmonary vascular disease, if the child survives infancy.

CLINICAL SIGNS

Bounding pulses, loud P2 and continuous or pansystolic murmur at mid- or lower left sternal edge. Large defects may have no murmur.

INVESTIGATIONS

- **ECG.** R and LVH.
- **CXR.** Cardiomegaly and pulmonary plethora.
- **Echocardiogram** is diagnostic but lesion can be missed, particularly if PDA coexists.
- **Cardiac catheterization** may be needed.

TREATMENT

Surgical correction at diagnosis, with high success rate.

Systemic arteriovenous fistula

INTRODUCTION

These are rare and may be single or multiple abnormalities. May occur at cerebral, coronary and hepatic sites.

NATURAL HISTORY

Large defects cause heart failure in infancy. Smaller shunts may not be of haemodynamic significance but may still be of local importance; for instance, intracerebral defects may cause cerebral ischaemia, hydrocephalus and fits without cardiac decompensation, and small coronary arteriovenous fistulae are risk lesions for endocarditis. A long-term risk of myocardial ischaemia in coronary arteriovenous fistulae exists.

CLINICAL FEATURES

Heart failure with bounding pulses may be present; a continuous bruit may be heard over the site (i.e. cranium, precordium or liver).

INVESTIGATIONS

- **ECG.** Right atrial enlargement, R and LVH.
- **CXR.** Cardiomegaly with or without pulmonary plethora.

- **Echocardiogram**. Volume-loaded right heart is found in significant lesions. An abnormal dilated coronary artery is often detectable and site of coronary arteriovenous connection found by colour flow Doppler. In intracranial lesions one of the aortic arch branches is usually large and SVC and right heart usually dilated.

TREATMENT

Heart failure therapy as indicated. If the shunt is of haemodynamic importance, catheter occlusion is preferred for intracranial shunts, surgery or catheter occlusion for coronary shunts and catheter occlusion, if possible, for hepatic lesions. Cerebral sequelae are not necessarily prevented by successful occlusion of intracranial malformations.

Obstructive lesions 16

INTRODUCTION

Aortic stenosis (AS)

Aortic stenosis can be at valvar, subvalvar or supravalvar levels in decreasing frequency and accounts for up to 5% of congenital heart disease. Bicuspid aortic valve can and often does exist without stenosis (see aortic regurgitation, Chapter 17, pp. 191–2). Valvar and subvalvar stenosis may exist in association with other left heart obstructive lesions and with VSD. Subvalvar obstruction may be discrete or diffuse (tunnel-like). Supravalvar aortic stenosis has a strong association with Williams syndrome (Chapter 3)

NATURAL HISTORY

Obstruction at any site may be progressive and may be associated with aortic regurgitation. Infants with severe AS may develop heart failure; the most extreme forms are critical AS and aortic atresia, which are lesions associated with duct-dependent systemic circulation. Aortic atresia is part of hypoplastic left heart syndrome (pp. 185–7). In older children with severe left ventricular outflow obstruction, near-syncope, syncope or chest pain on exertion are occasionally experienced.

CLINICAL FEATURES

Heart failure is present in severe/critical AS in infants. Pulses are weak in severe valvar stenosis; in supravalvar AS they may be full in the right arm, as a jet of blood is directed into the brachiocephalic trunk through the supravalvar aortic narrowing. A suprasternal thrill is often present; the apex may be forceful. Valvar AS is associated with an ejection click until it is severe; a harsh mid-systolic murmur is heard at the lower left sternal edge, aortic area and into the neck. There may be audible aortic regurgitation.

INVESTIGATIONS

- **ECG**
  - *Mild/moderate stenosis*: normal.
  - *Severe stenosis*: LVH by voltage criteria, with strain.
- **CXR**. Often normal. Pulmonary venous engorgement, cardiomegaly in symptomatic infants. Prominent ascending aorta.
- **Echocardiogram** is diagnostic. Left ventricular thickness and function can be assessed. Gradient can be estimated, usually with considerable accuracy, by Doppler.

TREATMENT

Intervention is indicated at any age if symptoms are present. Timing of treatment for asymptomatic individuals is influenced by age, speed of progression, associated lesions and the presence of ST/T changes on the ECG. Valvar stenosis is often managed by balloon dilatation although some centres prefer surgery, especially in early infancy. Neither surgery nor interventional catheter is curative and further treatment for residual/recurrent stenosis or for regurgitation is likely to be necessary eventually. Subvalvar and supravalvar stenosis have been treated by interventional catheterization but surgery is the usual approach. Mortality for all procedures is low except in critical AS in newborn infants.

Coarctation (CoA)   INTRODUCTION

Narrowing of the thoracic aorta at some point distal to the left subclavian artery occurs in up to 10% of congenital heart disease. The exact anatomical relationship to the ductus arteriosus varies and may have implications for the clinical presentation. Coarctation is commoner in males; in females the possibility of Turner's syndrome must be investigated by chromosome analysis even in the absence of other features. Bicuspid aortic valve occurs in two-thirds or more of cases of coarctation. Left ventricular outflow obstruction at other sites may coexist or develop; VSD is a common accompaniment. Coarctation may be a feature of more complex cardiac conditions, including TGA, double-inlet left ventricle and AVSD.

NATURAL HISTORY

Some cases of CoA may develop critical reduction in lower body blood flow when the ductus arteriosus shuts (there may be contractile ductal tissue in the aorta itself). These infants may present with collapse. In other cases heart failure will develop less dramatically in early infancy. Coexistent major lesions will affect the clinical picture and timescale of symptoms. Many cases remain asymptomatic until adverse effects of hypertension become apparent in the second or third decade, often in the form of cerebrovascular accident.

CLINICAL FEATURES

Collapse at the end of the first week of life will occur in one subset of patients; until resuscitated all pulses may be weak. Weak or impalpable femoral pulses in an infant with or without heart failure are diagnostic. Blood pressure is not necessarily elevated. A systolic bruit between the scapulae is usually present and in older children diastolic murmurs may be heard from collateral circulation. Signs of bicuspid aortic valve or other coexistent lesions are present. Upper and lower limb blood pressures may be helpful, but are not always reliable.

INVESTIGATIONS

- **ECG**
    - *Collapsed neonate*: RVH or normal.
    - *Older infant/child*: normal or LVH.
- **CXR.** Cardiomegaly if symptomatic. Pulmonary venous engorgement if symptomatic. Indentation lateral to the left upper mediastinal border (reverse E or 3 sign) may be seen. Rib notching is not seen until 8–10 years of age.
- **Echocardiography** is usually diagnostic but can be difficult in older children. Occasionally, cardiac catheterization or MRI is required.

TREATMENT

Resuscitation of a collapsed neonate specifically includes prostaglandin E_1 or E_2 prior to surgery. Intervention is also indicated if symptomatic or if hypertension or LVH is present. Mild coarctation occasionally causes none of these things, in which case careful surveillance is indicated until hypertension or LVH is documented. In older children exercise testing may reveal an excessive hypertensive response to exertion.

Surgery is generally preferred for native coarctation, although discrete localized lesions may be dilated by balloon catheter in selected cases even though the long-term results are usually better after surgery.

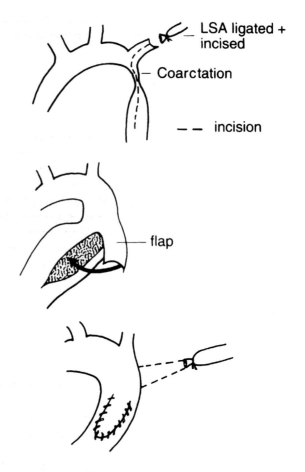

LSA ligated +
incised

Coarctation

— — incision

flap

Figure 16.1   Subclavian flap repair of coarctation. LSA = left subclavian
artery.

The left subclavian artery can be used for a subclavian flap aortoplasty
repair in the newborn and early infancy (Figure 16.1); the left arm pulse
is absent after this operation. End-to-end anastomosis after resection of
the coarcted segment is used in older children and is increasingly
popular in early infancy.

   Mortality for surgery is low unless other more complicated lesions
coexist, in which case coarctation repair is usually the first step or is
done simultaneously with intracardiac repair or pulmonary artery
banding. Recurrent or residual coarctation requires intervention in up
to 20% of postoperative cases; balloon dilatation is usually the treatment of choice.

   Hypertension is not necessarily abolished by treatment and continued
antihypertensive therapy is needed in some cases, particularly when

repair is carried out in later childhood or adult life. A proportion of patients will ultimately need aortic valve surgery, usually for aortic regurgitation.

Repair of coarctation in older children is associated with a small risk of paraplegia, particularly if there are few collateral vessels.

Interruption of the aortic arch

INTRODUCTION

This is much rarer than coarctation. There are several possible sites for the interruption but collapse when the ductus arteriosus closes is almost universal (Figure 16.2). Intracardiac abnormalities nearly always co-exist and include VSD, subvalvar left ventricular outflow obstruction, mitral stenosis and truncus arteriosus. There is a strong association with chromosome 22q11 deletions and DiGeorge syndrome.

NATURAL HISTORY

Survival beyond early infancy in untreated cases is very unusual; just occasionally the ductus arteriosus remains widely patent, when heart failure and failure to thrive are usually present; pulmonary vascular disease develops rapidly.

CLINICAL FEATURES

Collapse and gross heart failure are common. If examined before collapse, pulse differences around the arch (right arm, right side of neck, left side of neck, left arm, femorals) may allow the site of interruption to be determined. Physical signs of coexistent lesions may be apparent.

INVESTIGATIONS

- **ECG.** RVH.
- **CXR.** Cardiomegaly, pulmonary plethora; absent thymus in Di-George syndrome (not a sensitive sign).
- **Echocardiogram.** Diagnostic and allows further assessment of thymus.
- **Cardiac catheterization** is occasionally necessary for detailed delineation of anatomy.
- **Immune function** must be tested.

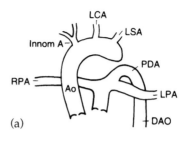

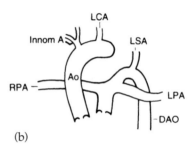

(a)

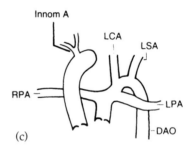

(b)

(c)

Figure 16.2 Types of interrupted aortic arch. (a) After left subclavian artery
(i.e. at isthmus of aorta). (b) Between the left carotid and left subclavian
arteries (the most common type). (c) Between the innominate and the left
carotid artery (very rare). Ao = ascending aorta; innom A = innominate
artery; LCA = left common carotid artery; LSA = left subclavian artery;
DAO = descending aorta; RPA = right pulmonary artery; LPA = left
pulmonary artery; PDA = patent ductus arteriosus.

TREATMENT

Initial specific resuscitation includes prostaglandin E_1 or prostaglandin
E_2. Surgical correction, with repair of intracardiac abnormalities if
possible, carries a mortality of 10–20%. Further surgery is often needed
for residual/recurrent arch obstruction and subvalvar left ventricular

outflow obstruction. Cellular blood products should be irradiated until immune status is known in case there is T-cell deficiency and a risk of graft *versus* host disease.

INTRODUCTION

This constitutes 3% of congenital heart disease. In its most typical form there is a small left atrium, an atretic mitral valve, a small left ventricle with thick walls and a tiny cavity and an atretic aortic valve. Thus pulmonary venous return passes through the foramen ovale into the right atrium and blood supply to the transverse and ascending aorta, including coronary arteries, is retrograde from the ductus arteriosus. There is frequently coarctation and in a few cases total anomalous pulmonary venous return.

Mitral atresia can occur without aortic atresia, usually in the context of double-outlet right ventricle; aortic atresia can occur without mitral atresia. In both these conditions there will occasionally be a sizeable VSD and two good-sized ventricles, which has implications for surgical strategies, particularly for aortic atresia without mitral atresia, when the possibility of establishing a two ventricle circulation exists.

NATURAL HISTORY

HLHS and aortic atresia without mitral atresia are fatal conditions when the ductus closes; this usually happens towards the end of the first week of life but it may be delayed, and survival to a few weeks or even a few months is occasionally seen. Mitral atresia without aortic atresia may be associated with longer-term survival.

CLINICAL FEATURES

Babies with HLHS are rarely completely well and usually have feeding difficulties from the start. However, they are often well enough to be discharged from maternity hospitals without a serious cardiac abnormality being suspected. Heart failure progresses rapidly and the baby will collapse when the ductus arteriosus closes. Before the ductus closes femoral pulses may seem stronger than upper limb pulses; once it has closed the baby will be tachypnoeic with massive hepatomegaly and impalpable peripheral pulses. There is frequently a gallop rhythm.

INVESTIGATIONS

- **ECG.** Right atrial enlargement, right axis deviation, RVH.
- **CXR.** Cardiomegaly, pulmonary venous engorgement; massive hepatomegaly often apparent.
- **Echocardiogram** is diagnostic.
- **Cardiac catheterization** is not necessary for diagnosis and carries a considerable morbidity and mortality.

TREATMENT

Babies with duct dependent systemic circulation are resuscitated with prostaglandin; some of these infants are critically ill and will require ventilatory support, diuretics and inotropes. Once stabilized, the options include:

- **Heart transplantation.** There are major problems with organ availability; quality of life can be good in the short and medium term but side effects from immunosuppression and acute and chronic rejection all complicate the outlook. Many families do not wish to pursue this path, even if a donor organ is available.
- Various **palliative procedures** have been developed, pioneered and refined, particularly by Norwood and colleagues. Essentially, the systemic outflow of the heart is recreated using the native pulmonary artery, and pulmonary blood supply is ensured by some form of systemic to pulmonary anastomosis. The second stage of the procedure involves establishing a Fontan-type circulation (total cavopulmonary connection). Some centres have achieved a 60–70% survival of the first stage and almost as good survival from the second, although many others have been unable to match this success rate. The procedure is regarded by many as buying time for transplantation: organs are more readily available for children of a few years of age and upwards. Variations on this approach have included transcatheter stenting of the ductus to stabilize systemic flow and banding of the pulmonary arteries with the ultimate goal of obtaining a transplant with fewer surgical interventions than the Norwood approach requires.

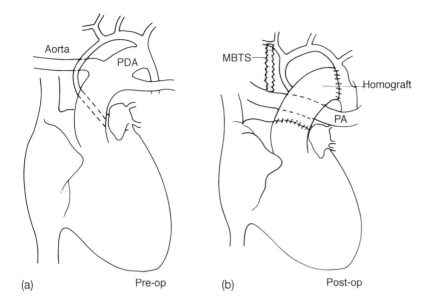

Figure 16.3   **Norwood operation for hypoplastic left heart.** (a) External appearance of heart before operation. (b) After operation. MBTS = modified Blalock–Taussig shunt; PA = pulmonary artery; PDA = patent ductus arteriosus.

- **No active treatment.** This is still a commonly followed approach but other options must be discussed fully and offered to families. Antenatal diagnosis is possible with ultrasound from around 18 weeks of gestation, and many parents decide not to continue with pregnancy.

INTRODUCTION

Pulmonary stenosis (PS)

This constitutes 8% of congenital heart disease and may be valvar, subvalvar or supravalvar. Valvar PS can be due to thin but fused valve cusps or thickened dysplastic cusps (often in association with Noonan's syndrome). Subvalvar PS is often associated with VSD, as in tetralogy of Fallot. Supravalvar stenosis can be in the main pulmonary artery or at the bifurcation or more distally. Williams syndrome, congenital rubella and Alagille's syndrome need to be thought of in children with pulmonary artery branch stenosis. Branch pulmonary artery stenosis can be iatrogenic after cardiac surgery, including systemic to pulmonary anastomoses, repair of tetralogy of Fallot or the arterial switch operation. All types of PS may be part of a more complex lesion, including TGA, tricuspid atresia and double outlet right ventricle.

NATURAL HISTORY

Progression may occur but mild/moderate valvar PS may never progress and pulmonary artery branch stenosis can improve with growth.

CLINICAL FEATURES

Critical valvar PS presents with cyanosis in the newborn period. Mild/moderate PS is asymptomatic in childhood. Severe PS may cause heart failure or effort-related dizziness or syncope. Clinical RVH and a thrill in the pulmonary area may be detected in moderate or severe cases; valvar PS will cause an ejection click until severe and a mid-systolic murmur in the pulmonary area also heard over the back and to the base of the left lung. Pulmonary artery branch stenosis causes a murmur laterally on the affected side(s).

INVESTIGATIONS

- **ECG**
  - *Mild stenosis*: normal.
  - *Moderate/severe stenosis*: progressively more marked RVH.
- **CXR**
  - *Mild stenosis*: normal.
  - *Moderate/severe stenosis*: dilatation of main pulmonary artery. RVH.
- **Echocardiogram.** Usually diagnostic and with Doppler studies allows gradient to be assessed accurately.

TREATMENT

Balloon dilatation is the treatment of choice for valvar PS and pulmonary artery stenosis (implantable stents may be needed with the latter). Treatment is indicated for symptoms and if RV pressure is more than 50% of systemic. Subvalvar stenosis is less successfully treated by catheter and surgery is generally used, as it is if balloon dilatation fails in valvar PS. Mortality is low for intervention of any kind (less than 3%).

Mitral stenosis (MS)   INTRODUCTION

This is a rare congenital lesion and usually accompanies (and may be masked by) other obstructive left heart lesions, ASD or VSD. Post-rheumatic MS remains common in many parts of the world, although often does not develop until later childhood or adult life.

NATURAL HISTORY

In congenital heart disease it is often determined by other lesions but pulmonary hypertension and right heart failure can develop.

CLINICAL FEATURES

A rumbling mid-diastolic murmur at the apex is a typical feature but may easily be masked or overlooked.

INVESTIGATIONS

- **ECG.** Left atrial enlargement, RVH.
- **CXR.** Large left atrium.
- **Echocardiogram** is usually diagnostic displaying valve anatomy well in young children. In older children transoesophageal echo may be helpful.
- **Cardiac catheterization** may be needed to assess pulmonary vascular resistance and in post-rheumatic MS may be used therapeutically for balloon dilatation.

TREATMENT

Surgery is generally required for symptomatic congenital MS or when right heart pressures are significantly raised. Coexistent lesions requiring surgery are likely to be present or to have required prior intervention. Balloon dilatation for post-rheumatic MS is widely used; it is rarely needed in young children.

Tricuspid stenosis

As a congenital lesion this accompanies other right heart abnormalities or is a feature of complicated lesions. It is very rarely the major lesion, when it is the picture would be that of tricuspid atresia (p. 207). Tricuspid stenosis can be a feature of Ebstein's anomaly, although tricuspid regurgitation is the more usual haemodynamic effect of this lesion (p. 194).

Regurgitant lesions 17

INTRODUCTION

Primary AR as congenital heart disease is usually due to a bicuspid aortic valve. Regurgitation may develop over time but not in all cases. AR can be secondary to endocarditis on a bicuspid valve, to valve distortion due to a cusp being drawn into a perimembranous VSD, to surgical or balloon treatment of aortic stenosis, to inflammatory processes (rheumatic fever, collagen vascular diseases) or to Marfan's syndrome in relation to aortic root dilatation. Symptomatic apparent AR in infancy is more likely to be due to aortico-left-ventricular tunnel than to true valvar AR.

NATURAL HISTORY

Structural abnormalities causing AR are likely to progress. Acute non-infective inflammatory causes of AR may improve if the process resolves. Infective endocarditis can cause rapidly fatal AR.

CLINICAL FEATURES

Bicuspid aortic valve and mild AR cause no symptoms. Breathlessness and heart failure occur with severe AR; chest pain may be experienced. Bicuspid aortic valve causes an ejection click at the lower left sternal edge and base. AR causes collapsing pulses, a dynamic precordium and suprasternal notch with displacement of the apex. An ejection click and mid-systolic murmur may be heard; a long, high-pitched, blowing diastolic murmur is best heard at mid- to lower left sternal edge. Sitting the patient forward facilitates auscultation. A rumbling mid-diastolic murmur may be heard at the apex from vibration of the anterior mitral leaflet in the regurgitant jet (Austin Flint murmur).

INVESTIGATIONS

- **ECG**
  - *Bicuspid aortic valve, mild AR*: normal.
  - *Moderate/severe AR*: LVH with strain.
- **CXR**
  - *Severe AR*: cardiomegaly, prominent ascending aorta.
- **Echocardiogram** usually displays anatomy and function well. Ventricular dimensions are important in assessing progress. Associated lesions must be sought (especially mitral regurgitation).
- **Cardiac catheterization** is rarely needed unless other lesions (including coronary artery disease in adults) need to be evaluated.

TREATMENT

Appropriate therapy for underlying diseases should be given. Anti-failure therapy should be instituted, if required, but symptoms are an indication for surgery. Echocardiographic demonstration of progressive left ventricular dilatation or deteriorating function are also indications for surgery. Valve replacement of some kind is indicated; artificial valves mean anticoagulation; homograft tissue valves are sometimes used. Placing the patient's own pulmonary valve and artery in the aortic position with a homograft in the pulmonary position (Ross operation) is used in some adolescents and young adults. The Ross operation has a higher mortality than valve replacement but is likely to last longer and does not require anticoagulation.

Mitral regurgitation (MR)

INTRODUCTION

Congenitally regurgitant mitral valves may have clefts or holes in a leaflet or leaflets may not coapt correctly. Mitral valve prolapse (MVP) may not cause regurgitation and is commonly not apparent until adolescence; it may develop in ASD and is seen in Marfan's syndrome. Mitral regurgitation is seen in AVSD and can be secondary to cardiac dilatation from any cause (such as heart muscle disease and volume overloading of the heart). MR is common in acute rheumatic fever; it often resolves but chronic rheumatic mitral valve disease may occur later in life.

NATURAL HISTORY

Progression in severity of MR may occur, although it is not invariable and the time-scale may be over years or even decades.

CLINICAL FEATURES

In childhood symptoms are rare; severe MR causes breathlessness. MVP is associated with supraventricular and ventricular arrhythmias. A mid- to late systolic click is the typical feature of MVP; there may be a late systolic murmur at the apex. The more severe MR will cause a dynamic precordium and a pansystolic murmur (sometimes with a thrill) at the apex.

INVESTIGATIONS

- **ECG**
  - *Mild/moderate MR*: normal.
  - *Severe MR*: LVH with strain.
- **CXR**
  - *Mild/moderate MR*: normal.
  - *Severe MR*: large left atrium.
- **Echocardiogram** usually delineates anatomy and cardiac dimensions well. Criteria for diagnosing mitral valve prolapse vary. A tiny amount of MR on colour flow Doppler is seen in many normal hearts.
- **Cardiac catheterization** is rarely needed.

TREATMENT

Arrhythmias and underlying diseases should be treated. Surgery is indicated for breathlessness or progressive dilatation of the left heart. Surgical repair of the valve is often possible initially, valve replacement may ultimately be necessary, prosthetic valves are always required and anticoagulation is essential.

Mitral valve prolapse

Mitral valve prolapse is extremely common, though the incidence varies in studies: it is probably found in approximately 1% of preschool children, but is more common in adolescents, with a prevalence of over 5% being recorded. The typical findings are a mid-systolic click and a late systolic murmur. Both may change with posture. The click and murmur are usually best heard at the apex. As with hypertrophic cardiomyopathy the murmur is loudest with standing and is quieter with squatting.

Morphologically the valve edges fail to oppose and the mitral valve billows into the left atrium. This is rather different from the flail mitral valve when the chordae are ruptured, for example after myocardial infarction. The diagnosis is established with two-dimensional echo-cardiography. Usually, antibiotic prophylaxis is required, although there is some controversy about the need for this. Mitral valve prolapse is associated with Marfan's disease, Ehlers–Danlos syndrome and a wide variety of congenital heart disease, and has been reported in association with many other conditions. Cardiological follow-up is advisable as arrhythmias have been recognized and, rarely, sudden death has been reported, which is presumably related to a ventricular arrhythmia.

Tricuspid regurgitation (TR)

INTRODUCTION

Tricuspid regurgitation due to structural congenital heart disease is usually due to Ebstein's malformation of the tricuspid valve, in which the septal leaflet is displaced towards the apex. Stenosis may result from this displacement but TR is the more usual lesion; an ASD is usually present. Ebstein's malformation often accompanies severe pulmonary stenosis and pulmonary atresia with intact ventricular septum. TR can be secondary to RV dysfunction after even fairly mild perinatal stress, and in association with severe pulmonary hypertension from any cause.

NATURAL HISTORY

Perinatal TR in structurally normal hearts resolves. When TR is secondary to other causes of RV hypertension the primary pathology determines natural history. The prognosis for Ebstein's anomaly is dependent on the severity of the lesion. Mild cases with minimal valve displacement are often asymptomatic; with severe Ebstein's there is gross displacement and a huge right atrium/atrialized right ventricle. The prognosis in the latter cases is poor.

CLINICAL FEATURES

Cyanosis will be present in severe Ebstein's anomaly (from right to left atrial shunting), with hepatomegaly, which may be pulsatile. S1 is widely split, with a loud tricuspid component; S3 and S4 are often heard, with a systolic murmur of varying length and intensity. Supra-ventricular arrhythmias are common with Ebstein's anomaly.

TR from other causes can be silent or cause a mid- or pansystolic murmur at the lower left sternal edge.

INVESTIGATIONS

- **ECG**
  - *Secondary TR*: abnormalities of underlying pathology.
  - *Ebstein's anomaly*: right atrial enlargement, pre-excitation, right axis deviation, small RV voltages.
- **CXR**
  - *Ebstein's anomaly*: right atrial prominence, huge heart in severe cases.
- **Echocardiogram** delineates anatomy well. Degree of regurgitation seen on colour flow Doppler. Many normal hearts have a tiny trace of TR.

TREATMENT

Arrhythmias should be treated appropriately. TR secondary to birth asphyxia or high right ventricular pressures require no specific treatment, although the underlying cardiac pathology may need treatment. Ebstein's anomaly may require tricuspid repair or replacement for severe TR and right heart failure. Decisions to close the ASD as well (or instead) can be difficult. If intervention is required in infancy for Ebstein's anomaly mortality is high.

Pulmonary incompetence (PI)

INTRODUCTION

PI can occur in pulmonary hypertension from any cause. It may also follow surgical relief of RV outflow obstruction, either valvar or subvalvar, and is typical of postoperative tetralogy of Fallot. Idiopathic dilatation of the pulmonary artery presents in the teenage years and is characterized by pulmonary regurgitation.

NATURAL HISTORY

PI will deteriorate in some cases but by no means all. In a few cases of postoperative PI a homograft valve may need to be inserted in the pulmonary position because of severe symptoms.

CLINICAL FEATURES

Symptoms may be due to underlying diseases; occasional idiopathic dilatation of the pulmonary artery with PI can cause breathlessness, reduced exercise tolerance and hepatomegaly. An abnormal valve or large pulmonary artery may cause an ejection click; there may be a quiet mid-systolic murmur in the pulmonary area and a high-pitched early to mid-diastolic murmur at the left sternal edge. In pulmonary hypertension the PI murmur may be mistaken for mitral stenosis (Graham Steell murmur).

INVESTIGATIONS

- **ECG**
  - *Severe PI*: RVH.
- **CXR** may show large central pulmonary artery.
- **Echocardiogram** is diagnostic; right heart dilatation is proportional to the severity of PI. Doppler studies help evaluate severity of PI. Colour Doppler is very sensitive and some degree of PI is present in many normal hearts.
- **Cardiac catheterization** may be needed to assess pulmonary vascular resistance.

TREATMENT

In severe cases (other than those secondary to pulmonary hypertension) pulmonary valve replacement is necessary.

Cyanotic lesions 18

There are three major categories of structural cyanotic congenital heart disease: some lesions can be classified into more than one category. The categories are:

- transposition of the great arteries;
- right-to-left shunt lesions;
- common mixing situations.

INTRODUCTION

Transposition of the great arteries (TGA)

Transposition exists when the aorta arises from the right ventricle and the pulmonary artery arises from the left ventricle. There are two forms of transposition.

Congenitally corrected transposition of the great arteries

In this very rare condition (< 1% of congenital heart disease) as well as the great arteries being transposed the atria are also connected in a discordant manner to the ventricles, i.e. pulmonary venous blood (saturated) flows through a morphological tricuspid valve into the right ventricle and systemic venous blood (desaturated) flows through a morphological mitral valve into the left ventricle. This arrangement will therefore not cause cyanosis unless coexisting abnormalities produce it, which they frequently do as VSD and important pulmonary outflow obstruction are often present.

Congenitally corrected transposition is often associated with Ebstein's anomaly of the tricuspid valve. This produces right ventricular to left atrial regurgitation, which will have the same haemodynamic consequences as mitral regurgitation would in a normally connected heart. Congenitally corrected transposition is associated with an increased tendency to supraventricular tachycardia and to complete heart block, which may be present at birth or may develop later.

This form of transposition is associated with clinical right ventricular hypertrophy, single S2 and appropriate murmurs if pulmonary stenosis or VSD or atrioventricular valve regurgitation are present. ECG will show complete heart block if present, marked right ventricular hypertrophy and strain and is particularly noteworthy for the presence of Q waves in the right chest leads and absence of them in V4–V6. The ECG will be further complicated if dextrocardia exists, which it does in a proportion of cases. Chest X-ray will show the heart position and often has a broad upper mediastinum because of the unusual relationship of the great arteries. Pulmonary vascular markings will be determined by coexistent lesions and the latter can be confirmed by echocardiography.

Surgical treatments are determined by the coexistent lesions but may involve VSD closure with relief of pulmonary outflow obstruction or systemic to pulmonary anastomoses and appropriate treatment of tricuspid regurgitation. Without coexistent lesions congenitally corrected transposition is associated with life into middle age or beyond but in most cases coexistent lesions will not allow this without surgical intervention.

Simple transposition of the great arteries

Simple transposition, i.e. without discordant atrioventricular connection, is the more usual form of transposition of the great arteries (TGA) and constitutes 5% of congenital heart disease. TGA is commonly associated with ASD, VSD and PDA and the degree of cyanosis will be determined by the number and size of shunt lesions. Clearly, some mixing is essential for postnatal survival; those infants depending only on a foramen ovale will be very blue from birth and become much bluer once the ductus arteriosus shuts. Coarctation can coexist. If there is left ventricular outflow obstruction, lung blood will be reduced and cyanosis more marked.

The site, nature and severity of LV outflow obstruction must be defined when planning surgical options, as discussed below. Transposition is only rarely associated with syndromes and extracardiac abnormalities.

The remarks in this section on transposition from now on only refer to this more common form of TGA.

NATURAL HISTORY

TGA without VSD presents with intense cyanosis in the early newborn period, made worse with rapid development of acidosis when the ductus arteriosus shuts or if the foramen ovale is severely restrictive. Similarly severe (usually subvalvar) pulmonary stenosis will cause intense early cyanosis made worse when the ductus shuts; these infants usually have VSD.

The presence of VSD without pulmonary stenosis or of a large PDA results in less marked desaturation and a later presentation, sometimes delaying diagnosis for weeks or occasionally months, when heart failure and failure to thrive have developed.

Survival beyond infancy without intervention is rare and only occurs in those with large VSD or PDA. Pulmonary vascular disease develops rapidly during infancy.

CLINICAL FEATURES

Early cyanosis and, particularly in those with shunt lesions, heart failure after some weeks are apparent. S2 is single because of the anterior position of the aorta and murmurs are unimpressive in simple TGA. If other lesions are present the relevant murmurs will be caused.

INVESTIGATIONS

- **ECG.** RVH. R and LVH if severe left ventricular outflow obstruction.
- **CXR.** Cardiomegaly, narrow superior mediastinum; pulmonary plethora unless severe pulmonary stenosis, when oligaemia is apparent.
- **Echocardiogram** is usually diagnostic and gives details of associated abnormalities.

TREATMENT

Resuscitation includes maintaining ductal patency with prostaglandin E series and balloon atrial septostomy (both improve mixing). Surgery to correct simple TGA and TGA with VSD is usually by the arterial switch procedure shortly after diagnosis. The great arteries are switched back to the appropriate ventricles, the pulmonary artery is usually brought forward anteriorly (Lecompte manoeuvre) and the coronaries are transferred with a button of aorta (Figure 18.1). Presentation after 3 weeks of age means that careful echocardiographic evaluation of the adequacy of the left ventricle to sustain systemic pressures is indicated (it usually becomes squashed and thin-walled as the pulmonary pressures fall to normal levels), but successful switch operations have been reported after 2–3 months. If doubt about the adequacy of the left ventricle exists, cardiac catheterization is needed and if necessary pulmonary artery banding is performed to prepare the left ventricle prior to the arterial switch procedure.

Mortality for arterial switch surgery is 10% or less, with a good long-term outlook. Some cases develop supravalvar pulmonary stenosis

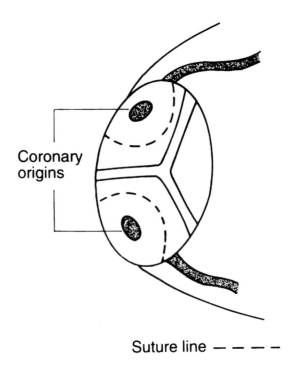

Coronary
origins

Suture line — — — –

**Removal of coronaries with "button"
from transected aorta**

Figure 18.1   Transfer of coronary arteries in the switch operation for
transposition.

requiring re-intervention. Intra-atrial repairs (Mustard or Senning operations) (Figure 18.2) are less favoured as long-term problems with
arrhythmias and poor right ventricular function become increasingly
apparent in young adults. TGA with VSD and severe left ventricular
outflow obstruction requires a systemic to pulmonary shunt initially,
with correction by VSD closure and some form of right ventricular to
pulmonary artery connection later in childhood, i.e. the Rastelli (Figure
18.3) (with pulmonary homograft) or REV (without homograft) procedure.

Right-to-left-shunts   INTRODUCTION

If there is obstruction to flow through the right heart with a natural
(patent foramen ovale) or abnormal (ASD, VSD) connection between

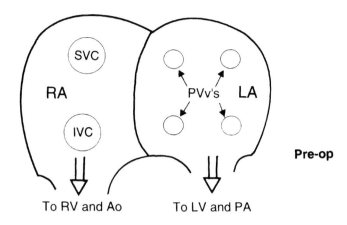

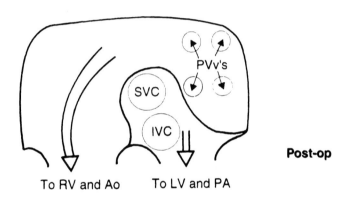

Figure 18.2 **Senning repair for transposition showing the atrial re-direction of venous flow.** SVC = superior vena cava; IVC = inferior vena cava; PVvs = pulmonary veins; Ao = aorta; PA = pulmonary artery; RV = right ventricle; LV = left ventricle.

right and left heart then varying quantities of desaturated systemic venous blood can avoid passage through the pulmonary vasculature and directly enter the systemic arterial circulation, resulting in cyanosis. The degree of arterial desaturation and other features will be determined by the severity of the obstruction and the size of the hole through which right-to-left shunting can occur. Lesions to be considered are:

- pulmonary stenosis and VSD (tetralogy of Fallot);
- critical pulmonary stenosis (with PFO or VSD);
- pulmonary atresia with intact ventricular septum;

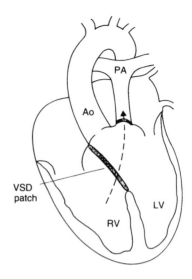

Direction of homograft tube

Figure 18.3   Rastelli repair of transposition/VSD pulmonary stenosis. The arrow shows the direction of the external conduit (see also Figure 18.9). RV = right ventricle; LV = left ventricle; PA = pulmonary artery; Ao = aorta.

- pulmonary atresia with VSD;
- tricuspid atresia.

TETRALOGY OF FALLOT

Introduction

(1) **Subvalvar pulmonary stenosis** due to anterior deviation of the infundibular ventricular septum, in association with (2) **an outlet VSD**, causes the aorta to arise partly from each ventricle (3) **overriding aorta** and, resulting in (4) **right ventricular hypertrophy**, constitutes tetralogy of Fallot (Figure 18.4), which accounts for 10% of congenital heart disease.

Valvar and supravalvar PS may also be present, as may right-sided aortic arch and, rarely, additional VSDs. Non-cardiac abnormalities are not uncommon, including chromosome abnormalities such as 22q11 deletions and Down's syndrome. Some cases of VSD may have coexisting valvar PS and some may develop muscular subvalvar RV outflow

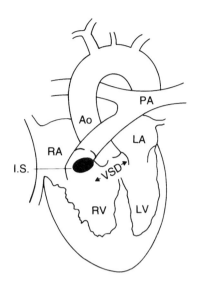

Figure 18.4   The anatomy of tetralogy of Fallot. 1. VSD. 2. Aorta (Ao) over-rides VSD. 3. Infundibular septum (I.S.) causes subpulmonary stenosis. 4. Right ventricular hypertrophy. PA = pulmonary artery; RA = right atrium; LA = left atrium; RV = right ventricle; LV = left ventricle.

obstruction; in either case haemodynamics become similar to tetralogy of Fallot, although the precise anatomy is somewhat different.

Natural history

A minority of cases of tetralogy of Fallot have very severe RV outflow obstruction or complete pulmonary atresia and they will be cyanosed as newborn infants. However, the majority are pink in the newborn period and subvalvar pulmonary stenosis progresses through infancy so that cyanosis is very common by 1 year of age. Survival to adolescence is unusual and it is rare to reach adult life; very occasionally, untreated middle-aged or elderly people with tetralogy of Fallot are encountered.

Clinical features

The progression of cyanosis is described above. Clubbing becomes apparent after infancy. Hypercyanotic spells may occur in infancy (p. 6). After infancy, squatting when resting after exertion may be seen; this is believed to increase systemic vascular resistance, thereby reducing intracardiac right-to-left shunting. It is not commonly seen, as the tendency to earlier intervention has resulted in fewer older children with marked cyanosis from tetralogy of Fallot. There may be a thrill in the pulmonary area, with a parasternal heave. P2 is quiet; there is a rough systolic murmur at the left upper sternal edge, which gets shorter as the right ventricular outflow obstruction progresses. There is no murmur from the VSD as it is large and ventricular pressures are equal. An ejection click may be present due to increased flow through the aortic valve in tetralogy of Fallot or through the pulmonary valve in cases of valvar pulmonary stenosis with VSD. An aortic regurgitant diastolic murmur may be heard in later childhood.

Investigations

- **ECG.** RVH.
- **CXR.** Prominent right ventricle, small central pulmonary arteries, pulmonary oligaemia; right aortic arch in 20%.
- **Echocardiography** is diagnostic.
- **Cardiac catheterization** is widely performed prior to corrective surgery and at times before palliation if pulmonary arterial abnormalities are suspected. Coronary artery anatomy, additional VSDs and pulmonary artery deformities are all relevant to surgical repair and can be defined angiographically.

Treatment

Surgical correction is achievable, with a 5% mortality or less in most cases in infancy or early childhood (Figure 18.5). Pulmonary atresia and pulmonary arterial abnormalities increase risk and make palliative systemic to pulmonary arterial shunts (e.g. Blalock) the initial procedure, with a view to correction later in childhood. A few cases have complicated pulmonary artery stenoses, for which transcatheter balloon dilatation and stenting is indicated, sometimes on several occasions. The long-term outlook for successful correction of uncomplicated cases is excellent, with a better than 90% 30-year survival, although some will have required further surgery for recurrent right ventricular outflow obstruction or progressive pulmonary regurgitation following surgery in early life.

Serious ventricular arrhythmias and progressive heart block can occur. Sudden death is recognized and is more common in those who had surgery later in childhood and in those who have important residual or recurrent haemodynamic disturbances. The role of detecting and treating ventricular arrhythmias in postoperative patients in an attempt to prevent sudden death is a matter for ongoing debate: if degrees of heart block progress postoperatively, pacemaker insertion is appropriate.

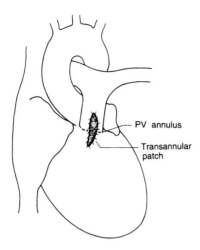

Figure 18.5   Tetralogy of Fallot. The external appearance of the heart when a transannular patch is used. In many cases, transannular incision is not needed and ventriculotomy (or atriotomy) may suffice. PV = pulmonary valve.

CRITICAL PULMONARY STENOSIS

Introduction

Severe pulmonary stenosis in the newborn results in tricuspid regurgitation and right-to-left shunting through the foramen ovale. Ductal closure may precipitate marked deterioration.

Natural history

Early death, either from profound hypoxaemia when the duct shuts or from heart failure, will occur.

Clinical features

Cyanosis and hepatomegaly will be present to varying degrees. P2 is inaudible; an ejection click is often not heard; pulmonary outflow murmur may be apparent, or a harsher murmur at lower left sternal edge from tricuspid regurgitation may be more prominent.

Investigations
- **ECG.** RVH.
- **CXR.** Right ventricular enlargement; pulmonary oligaemia.
- **Echocardiography** is diagnostic.
- **Cardiac catheterization** is not required for diagnosis.

TREATMENT

Cardiac catheter balloon valvuloplasty is usually possible; surgery also has a high success rate, with probably a lower rate for reintervention.

PULMONARY ATRESIA

Pulmonary atresia (when the pulmonary valve does not open at all thereby preventing any forward flow from the right ventricle to the pulmonary artery) can be subdivided into three groups.

1. Pulmonary atresia with intact ventricular septum (IVS)

This accounts for less than 1% of congenital heart disease and presents with cyanosis in the early newborn period that gets markedly worse when the ductus arteriosus shuts. The tricuspid valve is frequently abnormal and may be diminutive and stenosed.

The clinical picture is not unlike critical pulmonary stenosis except that no right ventricular outflow murmur is heard and the ECG has left axis deviation and LVH. Echocardiography allows a precise diagnosis but does not define the often present coronary artery abnormalities (sinusoids), which require angiography to be demonstrated well. However the value of this for decision making is disputed.

If at all possible surgical attempts to open the right ventricular outflow tract are appropriate. Interventional laser techniques are being evaluated. If the right ventricle is severely hypoplastic or outflow reconstruction is unsatisfactory in terms of relief of hypoxaemia, a systemic to pulmonary anastomosis is then indicated. Some patients are not suitable for biventricular repair and ultimately the establishment of a Fontan-type circulation is the goal.

Outcome is improving but survival to school age is only possible in approximately 75% of cases.

2. Pulmonary atresia with VSD without major sources of pulmonary blood flow other than PDA

These infants have duct-dependent pulmonary circulations and represent the severe end of the clinical spectrum of tetralogy of Fallot (see above).

3. Pulmonary atresia with VSD and important sources of lung blood flow other than PDA

These sources of lung blood flow are termed major aorto-pulmonary communicating arteries (MAPCAs). The pulmonary blood supply can be very complex: right and left pulmonary arteries may not be confluent and may not even exist.

The degree of cyanosis depends on the pulmonary blood flow and in some instances there may be excessive blood flow to the lungs or parts of them, causing pulmonary vascular disease. S2 is single; continuous murmurs are heard all over the chest. The ECG shows RVH and often LVH in addition; chest X-ray reveals cardiomegaly with a right ventricular contour, a small central pulmonary artery and often pulmonary plethora. Echocardiography does not define the pulmonary artery arrangement: angiography and/or MRI is required to do so.

Surgical options are individualized and may include shunting, attempts at repair in several stages involving drawing together all sources of lung blood flow (unifocalization), single stage repair and no intervention. Survival into adult life without intervention is known and surgical options need to be compared with the natural history.

TRICUSPID ATRESIA

Introduction

Absence or atresia of the tricuspid valve means that the only exit for blood from the right atrium is through a foramen ovale or ASD and is termed tricuspid atresia; it occurs in about 2% of cases of congenital heart disease. A VSD is almost invariably present. Associated abnormalities include pulmonary stenosis and transposition. Coarctation of the aorta may in addition be present in those with transposition.

Natural history

Those with either severe pulmonary stenosis or coarctation may be dependent on the ductus arteriosus and therefore collapse when it shuts. Those with transposition and those who have normally connected great arteries with a large VSD and no pulmonary stenosis will develop heart failure with high pulmonary blood flow, usually not until after the newborn period. If there is no transposition and the VSD is small, pulmonary oligaemia will result. Whatever precise anatomy exists, survival beyond infancy is very unusual without intervention.

Clinical features

Cyanosis is usually readily apparent even in those with high lung blood flow. S2 is single; a restrictive VSD may cause a harsh, long systolic murmur at the lower left sternal edge, whereas pulmonary stenosis will cause a mid-systolic murmur in the pulmonary artery. Signs of coarctation should be carefully sought and may be the presenting feature.

Investigations

- **ECG.** Right atrial enlargement, left axis deviation (usually about − 30°), LVH.
- **CXR.** Cardiomegaly, LVH. Pulmonary vascular markings reduced or increased according to haemodynamics.
- **Echocardiography** provides precise anatomical definition.
- **Cardiac catheterization** is not necessary for diagnosis but will be needed at a later stage for a haemodynamic assessment before definitive surgery of the Fontan type.

Treatment

Resuscitation with prostaglandin of the E series may be required. Coarctation if present should be repaired. If pulmonary oligaemia is present a systemic to pulmonary anastomosis (e.g. Blalock shunt) is appropriate to improve hypoxaemia. If lung blood flow is high pulmonary artery banding is indicated even if heart failure is absent or easily controlled, so as to protect against pulmonary vascular disease.

The long-term aim is to establish a Fontan-type circulation (total cavopulmonary connection) (Figure 18.6), in which systemic venous blood is directed in one or two stages (i.e. with a Glenn shunt first,

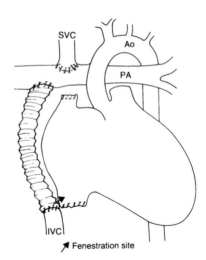

Figure 18.6   Total cavopulmonary connection with an extra cardiac conduit tube. Ao = aorta; PA = pulmonary artery; SVC = superior vena cava; IVC = inferior vena cava.

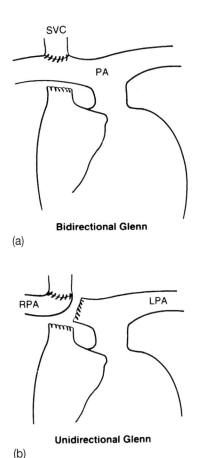

Figure 18.7   A Glenn shunt. (a) bidirectional; (b) unidirectional to right lung only. SVC = superior vena cava; RPA = right pulmonary artery; LPA = left pulmonary artery.

Figure 18.7) to the pulmonary arteries. Tricuspid atresia represents the best operative risk for such surgery (10% mortality) and the best long-term outlook (65% good-quality survival 10 years postoperatively).

Common mixing situations

Situations in which oxygenated and deoxygenated blood mix by mechanisms other than those already discussed under the heading of right-to-left shunts will result in systemic arterial desaturation. This may not necessarily be detected in the new born period if lung blood flow is unobstructed and therefore high. Conditions to be considered are:

- total anomalous pulmonary venous drainage;
- truncus arteriosus;

- univentricular atrioventricular connection;
- double-outlet ventricle.

TOTAL ANOMALOUS PULMONARY VENOUS DRAINAGE (TAPVD)

Introduction

This accounts for 1% of congenital heart disease. Drainage of the pulmonary veins can be:

- supracardiac (to SVC or innominate vein);
- cardiac (to right atrium or coronary sinus);
- infracardiac (to portal vein or IVC);
- mixed, if more than one form exists.

Atrial septal defect is an invariable accompaniment. VSD, PDA, coarctation and even hypoplastic left heart are occasionally found. The pulmonary veins can be obstructed at a number of sites and always are in infradiaphragmatic TAPVD. Pulmonary venous obstruction will cause more profound cyanosis and a smaller heart than unobstructed pulmonary venous pathways.

Natural history

Survival beyond infancy does not occur with obstructed TAPVD; it is not common, although it is well recognized, in unobstructed (usually supracardiac) TAPVD.

Clinical features

Cyanosis may not be detected until after the newborn period or can be intense and early, particularly in obstructed forms. In unobstructed TAPVD infants will sometimes present with apparent recurrent chestiness and failure to thrive. TAPVD to the portal vein is associated with severe obstruction when the ductus venosus closes. P2 will be loud and wide splitting of S2 is easily detected in those infants without obstructed veins, who often have a mid systolic murmur in the pulmonary area due to increased lung blood flow. Critically ill, very blue newborn infants with obstructed veins often have no murmurs and respiratory disease is frequently thought to be present.

Investigations

- **ECG.** Right atrial enlargement, right axis deviation, RVH.
- **CXR.** Cardiomegaly and pulmonary plethora if lung blood flow is high (pulmonary veins unobstructed). Broad upper mediastinum in

later infancy in supracardiac TAPVD (so called cottage loaf or snowman appearance). Small heart and opaque lung fields if pulmonary veins obstructed. In these circumstances X-ray changes are frequently mistaken for RDS with associated persistent pulmonary hypertension.
- **Echocardiography** is usually diagnostic, but ruling out the diagnosis in persistent pulmonary hypertension can be difficult as in both circumstances there is right-to-left flow across the foramen ovale. Precise anatomy can be difficult to obtain echocardiographically, particularly if mixed drainage sites exist.
- **Cardiac catheterization** is occasionally required to demonstrate anatomy adequately.

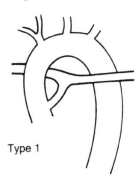

Type 1

Treatment

Prostaglandin is not generally indicated, nor beneficial, although occasional reports of improvement exist, related either to reopening the ductus arteriosus and subsequent decompression of the right heart or to opening the ductus venosus and alleviating pulmonary venous obstruction in infradiaphragmatic TAPVD. Obstructed TAPVD is one of the few conditions that is a surgical emergency and intense medical management is not likely to improve the infant's condition. In particular, infusions of colloid are badly tolerated and will not raise systemic blood pressure, which will be low because of poor pulmonary venous return. Corrective surgery has a mortality below 10% for most types, although severely obstructed pulmonary veins carry a greater risk. Providing severe left heart hypoplasia and pulmonary vein stenosis are not present, the long-term outlook is very good.

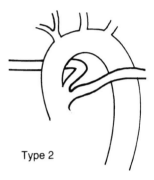

Type 2

TRUNCUS ARTERIOSUS

Introduction

This forms 1% of congenital heart disease and consists of a single arterial trunk leaving the heart that gives rise to aorta, coronary and pulmonary arteries. There is nearly always a very large VSD which the truncus overrides. Pulmonary artery attachments to the trunk vary (Figure 18.8); there may be a main pulmonary artery that divides (type I truncus), or each pulmonary artery may arise separately directly from the trunk, either adjacent to each other (type II truncus) or laterally from each side of the trunk (type III truncus).

Rarely, one pulmonary artery does not arise from the ascending trunk. Interruption of the aorta can occur. The truncal valve is abnormal and may have or develop important stenosis or regurgitation which

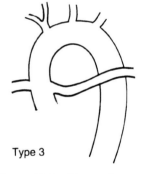

Type 3

Figure 18.8 Types of truncus arteriosus. The type is determined by pulmonary artery arrangement. Type 1: main PA arises from truncus, then divides. Type 2: right and left PAs arise adjacent to each other. Type 3: right and left PAs arise from each side of the truncus.

are both adverse prognostic features. There is a strong association with DiGeorge syndrome and 22q11 deletions, particularly so when aortic interruption coexists.

Natural history

Death in infancy is common but survival even to early adult life can rarely occur; in such circumstances pulmonary vascular disease is universal as significant pulmonary artery stenosis does not occur.

Clinical features

Heart failure with cyanosis is apparent but not necessarily until after the first few weeks of life. Pulses are usually bounding as there is marked run-off from the truncus/aorta into the pulmonary arteries. There is clinical RVH, an ejection click and a single S2. A pansystolic murmur at the lower left sternal edge, if heard, is likely to be due to tricuspid regurgitation rather than the VSD, as the defect is almost invariably large and ventricular pressures are equal. Truncal valve stenosis and regurgitation sound like the equivalent aortic murmurs. A rumbling apical mitral diastolic murmur may be heard as a manifestation of high pulmonary blood flow.

Investigations

- **ECG.** Right axis deviation, RVH with or without LVH.
- **CXR.** Cardiomegaly, pulmonary plethora; right aortic arch may be present.
- **Echocardiography** is diagnostic.
- **Cardiac catheterization** is only needed if pulmonary artery anatomy needs to be further defined, when **MRI** may be both better and safer than catheterization. Cardiac catheterization to assess pulmonary vascular resistance may be indicated in late presenting cases, when the question of whether they are still operable needs to be considered.

Treatment

Corrective surgery is appropriate in early infancy. Some form of conduit from right ventricle to pulmonary artery is required (Figure 18.9) and later replacement is very likely to be needed. Mortality is less than 20% unless severe truncal valve regurgitation or aortic interruption is present, when risks are considerably higher. Pulmonary artery banding as

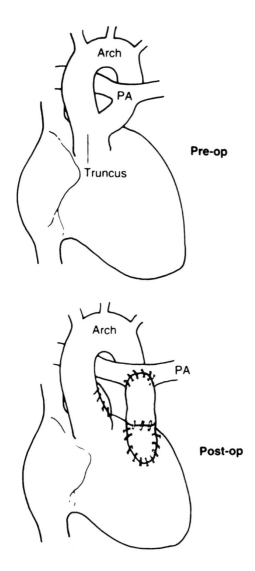

Figure 18.9   The technique of using a homograft to connect the right ventricle to pulmonary arteries in truncus arteriosus. The VSD is closed through a ventriculotomy. PA = pulmonary artery.

initial palliation is no longer favoured. Blood products should be irradiated until T-cell numbers are known because of the possibility of DiGeorge syndrome (p. 38) and the risk of graft *versus* host disease.

UNIVENTRICULAR ATRIOVENTRICULAR CONNECTION (DOUBLE INLET VENTRICLE, SINGLE VENTRICLE)

Introduction

This group of abnormalities used to be called single ventricle, which description does convey the common mixing of saturated and desaturated blood that occurs. The presence and size of a VSD (there is usually a second, rudimentary ventricle) and the great artery arrangements will determine the overall clinical picture. Double inlet ventricle is most usually of left ventricular morphology; the great arteries may be transposed and there may be either systemic or pulmonary outflow obstruction but very rarely both.

Natural history

Prolonged survival without intervention can occur in occasional cases but this is not generally the rule.

Clinical features

These complicated lesions may present early if there is either duct-dependent pulmonary or systemic circulation (p. 76). Heart failure will occur in those with no significant pulmonary outflow obstruction; cyanosis will be milder in these cases. Cyanosis is more obvious in those with valvar or subvalvar pulmonary stenosis.

Investigations

- **ECG.** Rarely normal; left or right atrial and ventricular forces may be abnormal.
- **CXR.** Rarely normal. Cardiomegaly and pulmonary plethora if high pulmonary blood flow. Normal heart size and pulmonary oligaemia if pulmonary stenosis. Abnormality of heart position may be present.
- **Echocardiography** usually clarifies detailed anatomical and haemodynamic information. Cardiac catheterization is needed before certain treatment options are embarked on, particularly prior to establishing a Fontan circulation.

Treatment

Corrective surgery in establishing a biventricular circulation is rarely possible. Palliative interventions may be indicated in early infancy in the form of repair of coarctation, if present, pulmonary artery banding for high pulmonary blood flow and systemic to pulmonary anastomosis (e.g. Blalock shunt) for pulmonary oligaemia. The long-term objective for many is the establishment of a partial (Glenn shunt) or total (Fontan circulation) cavopulmonary connection. There are many contraindications and additional risk factors for this approach. The long-term outlook is best for those with a morphologically left ventricle as the systemic ventricle.

DOUBLE OUTLET VENTRICLE

Introduction

When both great arteries arise chiefly from one ventricle the term double outlet ventricle is used. Double outlet right ventricle is far more common than double outlet left ventricle. Double outlet right ventricle (DORV) can be associated with mitral atresia. In DORV with normal atrioventricular connections the great artery arrangements determine the clinical picture. If the pulmonary artery is posterior and overrides a VSD the haemodynamics are very similar to TGA with VSD. If the pulmonary artery is anterior and the VSD is nearer the aorta the clinical picture will resemble a large VSD if there is no pulmonary stenosis, and tetralogy of Fallot if there is valvar or subvalvar pulmonary stenosis. DORV with subpulmonary VSD and an anterior aorta may be associated with coarctation. DORV can be associated with very complex CHD, as in atrial isomerism.

Natural history

This will be determined by the presence or absence of VSD and pulmonary stenosis or atresia. Occasionally, long-term survival without intervention is possible but most infants will be symptomatic at an early stage and have limited life expectancy without surgical intervention.

Clinical features

These are determined by coexistent lesions and may resemble transposition, VSD or tetralogy of Fallot.

Investigations

- ECG. Very rarely normal except in the early newborn period.
- CXR. Cardiomegaly with pulmonary plethora, or normal heart size and pulmonary oligaemia are the two characteristic appearances.

- **Echocardiography** usually delineates anatomy accurately without the need to proceed to cardiac catheterization.

Treatment

Surgical treatment will consist of repair in some circumstances and palliative procedures with a view to later repair in others.

Miscellaneous cardiac and cardiorespiratory disorders 19

Cardiac tumours

Cardiac tumours are uncommon. The most frequent tumour in the paediatric age group is a rhabdomyoma. Usually this is associated with tuberous sclerosis and if there is more than one rhabdomyoma then it seems almost certain that the child has tuberous sclerosis. Often the diagnosis is made in fetal life and there is a period of rapid tumour growth during the last trimester. The tumours can regress during infancy and therefore surgery is not indicated unless the tumour is causing significant obstructive symptoms. Sometimes the rhabdomyoma can irritate the myocardium and cause a ventricular tachycardia, or may act as an accessory pathway and cause a supraventricular tachycardia.

Teratomas are occasionally seen in children. Usually, they are intra-pericardial and attach to the arteries at the base of the heart. Fibromas have also been recorded and may be difficult to resect completely. Haemangiomas and myxomas are uncommon in children and primary and secondary malignant tumours are rare in the paediatric age groups. Some benign tumours have been reported in the conduction tissue and they can lead to heart block or intractable arrhythmias; these may include mesothelioma of the atrioventricular node and Purkinje hamartoma.

Vascular rings

Vascular compression of the trachea (vascular ring) may cause stridor in infancy. This characteristically has an expiratory component and in most cases is present from the early neonatal period. Associated cardiac anomalies occur in approximately 10% and these are typically either a VSD or a conotruncal abnormality (e.g. Fallot's tetralogy, truncus arteriosus, pulmonary atresia with ventricular septal defect). The majority of vascular rings are caused by a double aortic arch (60–70%; Figure 19.1).

The next most common lesions are pulmonary artery sling in which the left pulmonary artery arises from the right pulmonory artery (10–20%) and right aortic arch with an aberrant left subclavian and a

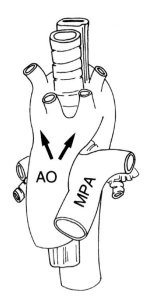

Figure 19.1   Double aortic arch, viewed from the front. AO = ascending aorta; MPA = main pulmonary artery; arrows show the bifurcation of the aorta into right and left arches, which then encircle the trachea and oesophagus.

left duct or ligament (10–20%). Occasionally there may be a right aortic arch with a left retro-oesophageal duct or ligament. Rarely there may be a left aortic arch with right descending aorta and a right duct or ligament, the importance of this abnormality being that a right thoracotomy must be used to ligate the ligament and relieve the compression whereas the other abnormalities can be repaired by a left thoracotomy (although occasionally a median sternotomy is required for a pulmonary artery sling because of extensive reconstructive work required to the pulmonary arteries and often the trachea).

Severe tracheal anomalies are more common with pulmonary artery slings, when there may be complete cartilaginous rings in the trachea. Also pulmonary artery slings are occasionally associated with hypoplasia of one lung and subsequent mediastinal shift. An isolated aberrant right subclavian artery passing posterior to the oesophagus does not cause a vascular ring unless there is a duct or ligament from the aberrant subclavian. Aberrant subclavian arteries usually cause no symptoms at all, although they could conceivably result in dysphagia. In most cases they are an incidental finding.

Potentially an iatrogenic ring could be constructed by connecting a modified Blalock shunt between an aberrant subclavian artery and the pulmonary artery, although, in the cases where this has been performed, there is rarely any compression. An anomalous origin of the innominate artery has also been listed as a cause of vascular rings but innominate origin to the left of the trachea is common in normal subjects and it seems much more likely that the obstructive symptoms relate to a localized area of primary tracheomalacia and the pulsatile compression seen anteriorly at bronchoscopy reflects this tracheomalacia rather than any anomalous origin of the innominate. This lesion may be relieved by aortopexy.

INVESTIGATIONS

Assessment for a child with stridor from a suspected vascular ring should include a barium swallow. False-positive diagnoses are rare and false-negative diagnoses are uncommon. Therefore, barium seems to be the ideal screening test for vascular rings. Pulmonary artery slings typically cause an anterior compression whereas a double aortic arch will show bilateral indentation, which is often most obvious in oblique and lateral views (Figure 19.2). An aberrant subclavian artery causes a posterior indentation.

Once there has been a positive barium swallow the best investigation to define the anatomy is echocardiography with colour flow Doppler. Angiography and MRI may require sedation and/or ventilation and probably neither is superior to echocardiography.

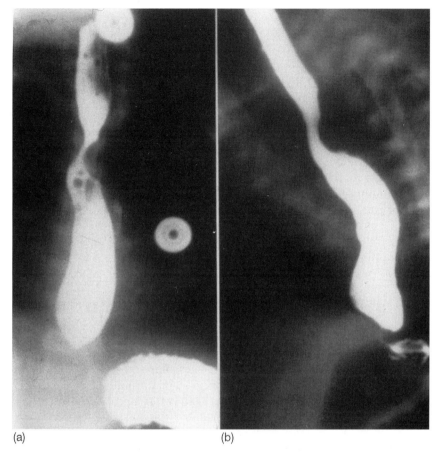

(a)   (b)

Figure 19.2   Barium swallow showing bilateral indentations on the antero-posterior view (**a**) and a marked posterior indentation on the lateral view (**b**). Double aortic arch. From Burch, M. *et al.*, *Arch Dis Child*. 1993; 68: 171–177, by kind permission of BMJ Publishing Group.

Cor pulmonale

This is cardiac disease induced by an airway or lung disorder. The cardiac problem is right ventricular hypertrophy, dilatation or failure. There is pulmonary artery hypertension, which is often induced by chronic hypoxia. An elevated CO_2 will also affect pulmonary arterial resistance, as will polycythaemia.

A common cause of chronic hypoxia and hypercapnia in children is upper airway obstruction. This is most obvious at night and there is often a history of sleep disturbance and snoring. Children with Down's syndrome may have quite marked upper airway obstruction, which can accelerate the rate of development of pulmonary vascular disease in those children with an associated cardiac septal defect. Children with the Robin anomaly or macroglossia may also have severe airway

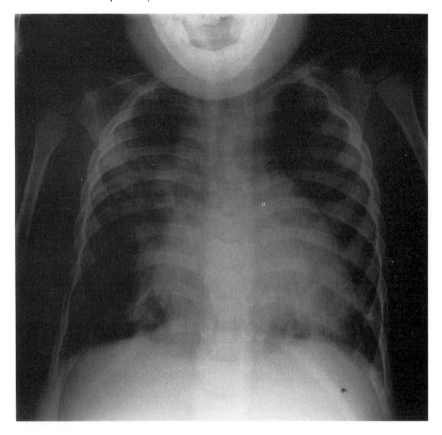

Figure 19.3   Postero-anterior chest X-ray showing cardiomegaly with a prominent right atrium, overinflated lung fields with widespread patchy changes. Cor pulmonale in a 2-year-old with chronic lung disease related to prematurity and previous VSD (surgically closed).

obstruction. Occasionally the obstruction may be laryngeal from laryngotracheomalacia. In many cases, the tonsils and adenoids are hypertrophied and their removal can improve symptoms. Sometimes a nocturnal airway is used and occasionally tongue reduction is needed. The diagnosis of upper airway obstruction is usually made during sleep study where oxygenation, respiratory pattern, heart rate and sometimes CO_2 can be monitored during sleep.

Bronchopulmonary dysplasia may cause cor pulmonale (Figure 19.3), but cardiac problems are uncommon in paediatric patients with cystic fibrosis and restrictive lung disease (a well recognized cause of cor pulmonale in adults) is uncommon in children.

Neuromuscular diseases, scoliosis and central hypoventilation have also been documented as causing cor pulmonale. Pulmonary emboli can also cause right heart failure in an acute or chronic form. They are rare in children, but have been documented in patients with central venous lines (for example those on home parenteral nutrition) and after cardiac surgery.

Treatment is usually aimed at the cause of the pulmonary hypertension and hypoxia should be treated.

Scimitar syndrome

In the full scimitar syndrome there is dextrocardia because of hypoplasia of the right lung and right pulmonary artery, anomalous pulmonary venous drainage of some (or all) of the right-side pulmonary veins to the inferior vena cava, and an abnormal arterial supply to the right lower lobe from the aorta below the diaphragm. The term 'scimitar' was used because of the sword-like appearance of the abnormal venous drainage on the chest X-ray.

Sometimes there is associated congenital heart disease. Often patients are reasonably well balanced but if they are symptomatic surgery is indicated.

Some children have an isolated anomalous arterial supply to the lung which is described as a sequestration and is usually to the left and posteriorly. Sometimes there is no connection of the pulmonary tissue to the airways. These patients tend to present with recurrent infections of the sequestrated lobe although sometimes there are no symptoms. Surgery is indicated in symptomatic patients.

Absent pulmonary valve syndrome

With this abnormality there is an abnormal pulmonary valve ring with free pulmonary regurgitation and severe pulmonary stenosis and typically a 'Fallot' type of VSD. There is usually gross dilatation of the pulmonary arteries which results in tracheobronchial compression and subsequent pulmonary symptoms. Surgical treatment is difficult and carries a significant risk.

Pulmonary arteriovenous malformations

These lesions are often asymptomatic initially but may present with haemoptysis or progressive cyanosis. The diagnosis is established using digital subtraction angiography or CT or MRI scanning.

Multiple anomalies and lung defects may be associated with hereditary haemorrhagic telangiectasia. Sometimes they may be associated with structural congenital heart disease, for instance, left isomerism or they may develop in some patients after cardiac surgery, typically those in whom a passive filling pulmonary circulation (Fontan circuit) has been created. Pulmonary arteriovenous malformations have also been found to be associated with liver disease.

Treatment is now by interventional cardiac catheterization with coil occlusion of the abnormalities. Often multiple procedures are required and new malformations can develop with time.

Pulmonary hypertension

Primary pulmonary hypertension is rare in children, but paediatricians will occasionally see cases and some may be familial. Onset in infancy is usually associated with a rapid deterioration, with development of right heart failure and death in early childhood. Some children may survive for a longer period.

Treatment is very difficult, but long-term calcium channel antagonists can be beneficial. Oral anticoagulants and treatment with oxygen can be helpful in selected cases. Intravenous prostacyclin has been used in adults. Ultimately these patients may need heart–lung transplantation.

Kartagener's syndrome

The dextrocardia and situs inversus of Kartagener's syndrome is inherited as a recessive trait. The main respiratory problem is cilial dyskinesis, which results in chronic chest infections. These patients need advice about home physiotherapy and appropriate antibiotic treatment of chest infections. Septal defects and other cardiac abnormalities are associated, but many cases have no structural cardiac defect other than dextrocardia.

Pulmonary venous obstruction

Rarely there may be severe pulmonary venous obstruction either at the origin with the left atrium or over an extended length (hypoplasia). This can present neonatally or can be a progressive condition. The prognosis is very poor and surgical treatment is not usually possible.

Recommended further reading

Allan, L. D., Sharland, G. K. and Cook, A. C. (1994) *Colour Atlas of Fetal Cardiology*, Mosby-Wolfe, London.

Burch, M. (1996) *Oxford Paediatric Echocardiography Course Video*, Oxford Medical Illustration, Oxford.

Emmanouilides, G. C., Riemenscheinder, T. A., Allen, F. I. D. and Gutgesell, H. P. (1995) *Heart Disease in Infants, Children and Adolescents*, 5th edn, 2 vols, Williams & Wilkins, Baltimore, MD.

Gillette, P. C. and Garson, A. (1990) *Pediatric Arrhythmias: Electrophysiology and Pacing*, W. B. Saunders, Philadelphia, PA.

Ho, S. Y., Baker, E. J., Rigby, M. L. and Anderson, R. H. (1995) *Colour Atlas of Congenital Heart Disease*, Mosby-Wolfe, London.

Kirklin, J. W. and Barratt-Boyes, B. G. (1993) *Cardiac Surgery*, 2nd edn, 2 vols, Churchill Livingstone, Edinburgh.

Park, M. K. and Guntheroth, W. O. (1992) *How to Read Pediatric ECGs*, 3rd edn, Year Book, Chicago, IL.

Perloff, J. K. (1987) *The Clinical Recognition of Congenital Heart Disease*, 3rd edn, W. B. Saunders, Philadelphia, PA.

Silverman, N. H. (1993) *Pediatric Echocardiography*, Williams & Wilkins, Baltimore, MD.

Index

Page numbers appearing in **bold** refer to figures.